TRAVELING ON THE RIVER OF DEMENTIA

A Family's Perspective

PATRICIA M. BUTLER

Copyright@ 2025 Patricia M. Butler

All rights reserved. No part of this publication may be reproduced, stored or transmitted in any form or by any means, electronic, mechanical, photocopying, recording, scanning, or otherwise without written permission from the publisher. It is illegal to copy this book, post it to a website, or distribute it by any other means without permission, except in the case of brief quotations embodied in critical reviews and certain other noncommercial uses permitted by copyright law.

Printed in the United States of America

100% Human Generated Content

Library of Congress Control Number: Txu 2-488-955
Paperback ISBN: 979-8-218-67637-7
Ebook ISBN: 979-8-218-67638-4

Cover design by Marjorie Daley
Book design and production by Marjorie Daley
Cover photograph by Patricia M Butler

For bulk orders, contact the author at
patriciambutlerauthor@yahoo.com

Images of Dementia
Allegories, similes, and metaphors,
Like a poem, without meter or rhyme

For my family
and
all those traveling on the river of dementia

Dear Reader,

This is a story of my family's journey along the river of dementia. It is a story of my mother's travels through the waters, my father's love and devotion while on the river with her, my sister's joys and pains negotiating the currents, and my thoughts while watching from the banks and giving navigational directions from a distance.

It is also a crazy quilt of my mother's life, a crazy quilt made up of bits and pieces, scraps and patches, all put together with threads of love. It is a beautiful crazy quilt of a wonderful life spanning over 98 years, 68 wedding anniversaries, two daughters, four grandchildren, and 5 great-grandchildren.

I hope these pieces will honor my mother's life and my family's voyage on this river. I hope it will give solace and hope and an understanding of the dementia process to others involved with their own stories. It is not a finished piece yet. My mother continues to be swept downward on the river of dementia, and the quilt is not finished yet, not yet.

We as a family and individually are growing in understanding of her memory loss and behaviors. We hope to continue the journey with greater insight and greater love. We will be with her until she disembarks at her final destination. We will be with her until the quilt is completed, the last thread is stitched.

May you find a deeper level of understanding as you travel on that river of dementia, and may you find beauty in all the bits and pieces of your own crazy quilt.

Patricia M. Butler

INTRODUCTION

I have been dealing professionally with dementia and especially Alzheimer's Disease for over 28 years. I was part of the team that opened the first Special Care Unit for the care and treatment of Alzheimer's Disease in the state of Wyoming. My team gave workshops throughout the state, educating the public and professionals about Alzheimer's Disease and how to provide the best care. I served on the State of Wyoming Alzheimer Association Board and also served as its Chairperson.

As an Alzheimer's Support Group facilitator for over 28 years, I have gained the expertise to help people with Alzheimer's Disease and related dementias. I have learned from the personal stories of families and friends of those with dementia. Whatever understanding I have comes from my professional training, my work with families in the support groups, my work at the nursing home, and my personal experiences with my family. Having expertise to help people with dementia does not take away the agony and pain, frustrations and uncertainties, I feel in dealing with my mother and our family. It is my hope you will come to understand some of our feelings and the issues regarding my mother's and our family's personal journey. I hope you will learn from our story and come to understand more clearly the enigma of dementia.

TABLE OF CONTENTS

FROM LIGHT INTO DARKNESS INTO LIGHT	1
UMOR	2
RIDING THE RIVER	3
WYOMING STYLE	5
FLYING OVER THE LARAMIE RIVER	6
CRAZY QUILT	7
GOING CRAZY	12
READING	13
LISTEN	14
ARE YOU LISTENING	15
TRIP TICS	16
TRAVELING ON	18
VACATIONS	19
A FARAWAY PLACE	20
PIANO	21
DO YOU HAVE THE TIME	22
MEMORIES	25
WHAT ARE THOSE LADIES SAYING ABOUT ME	26
FOR BETTER OR WORSE	27
DO YOU STILL LOVE ME	28
FOG	29
THERE'S SOMEBODY HERE	30
JUMBLE	31
HIDING	32
DANCE WITH ME	33
FIND ME MY MEMORY	34
TIME	35
MISS YOU	36
BAKING	37
NO MORE BAKING	39
SHE LOST HER MEMORY	40
MY SISTER	41

SISTER IS UP CLOSE AND PERSONAL	42
AT A DISTANCE	44
TIDBITS	45
DOWNSIZING STUFF	46
NOT DONE	48
STUFF	49
MY SEWING MACHINE	50
SEWING MACHINE	51
INCONTINENCE	53
LOST CONTROL	54
DRESSING UP	55
ALL DRESSED UP	56
COOKING	57
THE COOK IS DONE	58
STARVING	59
MORE CALCIUM	60
LIFESAVERS	61
SWIMMING	62
MEMORIES	64
CHURCH	65
GOD AND ME	67
LONELY	68
LONELINESS	69
HOME AGAIN	70
HOME	71
SLIP SLIDING AWAY	72
THE BUS	73
MOTHER LOVE	74
PRISONER	76
EYES	77
FORK IN THE RIVER	79
RUST	80
GOODBYE	81
A LITTLE BIT OF DYING	82
WATER	83

FLOATING AWAY	85
FLOWING, FLOATING, OR DROWNING	86
TEA	87
SWEETNESS	89
MEDS	90
CAN HE STILL DO IT	91
ENERGIZER BUNNY	93
ON THE MOVE	94
WE BOTH HURT	95
NO ROOM	96
DAM HAS BROKEN	97
DROWNING	98
WINTER IS COMING	99
NO LONGER HERE	100
GRANDMA AND GRANDPA	101
RAINBOW	103
TIDBITS	104
DARKNESS	105
LIGHTNING	106
MORE THAN THEY CAN HANDLE	107
DEEP WATER	108
PRAYER	109
THERE IS ROOM AT THE INN	110
SHE'S CHANGED	111
I'VE CHANGED	112
RELIEF	113
TIDBITS IN HUNGARIAN	114
ADMIRATION FROM A SON-IN-LAW	115
MY RELIEF	116
SEPARATE BUT NOT APART	117
LOCKED AND UNLOCKED	118
DON'T LEAVE ME ALONE	119
I DON'T WANT TO BE ALONE EITHER	120
ACCEPTING THE UNACCEPTABLE	121
THE DOCTOR	122

THE PAID CAREGIVERS	123
DON'T LIKE IT HERE	125
COMMUNICATION	126
COME ON IN, THE WATER'S FINE	127
CHIPPER MOM	128
A GLORIOUS DAY	129
THE DANCE: A WALTZ IN ¾ TIME	130
JITTERBUGS	132
KARAOKE	134
LESSONS TO LEARN	135
BENEDICTIONS	136
FOG HAS SETTLED IN	137
FILL YOUR POT	138
THOUGHTS WHILE RETURNING ON THE PLANE	139
BUMPY RIDE	140
MY SEPARATION	141
IN THE MIDST OF THE WHIRLWIND	142
A SHIFT	144
CHECKING UP AFTER THE TORNADO	145
SHUFFLING OFF	147
AFTER FALLING OFF THE BUS	148
SHE'S NOT HERE, DAD'S LAMENT	149
SHE'S EDGY AND HE STILL LOVES HER	151
MOTHER'S DAY	153
HE JUST KEEPS ON KEEPING ON	154
DOWN THE HIGHWAY FOR A WALK	155
DEPENDS	156
DAD'S BIG THREE	158
THE SECOND THING I MISS	159
NUMBER THREE TO DEAL WITH	161
GOING DOWNHILL	162
SHE WON'T LET ME IN	164
HOW CAN IT BE LIKE THIS	166
HURRICANES	167
DAD IS FIGHTING THE CURRENT	168

FALLING BACKWARD	169
FALLING	170
SISTER IS FALLING	171
FULL BODY ARMOUR	173
WITHDRAWAL	174
MOM'S HANDS	175
GREATER OR LESSER, THEM OR THOSE PEOPLE: IT DEPENDS ON YOUR VIEW	178
HE NEEDS TO DRINK, DRINK, DRINK	180
ICE AGE	182
BOULDERS AND SNAGS	183
ODE TO MY SUPPORT GROUP	184
I DON'T LIKE THE WATER	186
ROLLING ON THE RIVER	187
THE CANE	188
BRIDGES	189
UNDERCURRENTS	190
OUT OF CONTROL	191
WAITING FOR THE WELCOMING PARTY	192
WHO WILL GO FIRST?	193
PLAN B	194
PRACTICING FOR THE FINAL	195
IS THERE LIFE AFTER CAREGIVING?	196
HE WENT FIRST	197
FINAL JOURNEY	202
FINAL GOODBYE	204
SIX YEARS LATER	205
IT'S OVER	206
WHEN IT'S OVER	208
THE RIVER OF TIME	209

FROM LIGHT INTO DARKNESS INTO LIGHT

Traveling along the river of dementia
is like traveling through a barren landscape.
We go from light to darkness.
In the beginning God created light out of darkness,
out of the dark void.

This disease is the opposite.
We start out in the full blazing light of knowledge,
of joy, of illumination.
It's as if the light of reality dims,
and the person goes into the darkness of loss.
The mind's memory fades and grays
until the light goes out.

Occasionally the sun peeks through,
a moment of time is saved and savored.
Then the clouds come back,
and the darkness takes over.

I know in time there will be no more sun,
no more time for Mom.
When she goes, will our light go out too?

At the end of her journey
she will enter the fullness of a new life,
filled with the light of God.

No darkness for us on this river.
We will be lit by the joyous memories of times gone by,
by the illuminating smiles of past remembrances.
We may need a flashlight on this journey.

I hope our batteries hold up.

UMOR

Definition of Humor - fluid, like water, from the Latin word 'umor'

We need a sense of humor dealing with Mom and Dad.
We need to be more relaxed during the stressful times.
We need to be more fluid and flexible.

Sometimes we feel so breakable in the face of
the relentless change.
We need this 'umor' to help us flow through the difficulties,
instead of being swamped by them.

As we travel along this river of dementia,
may we find the water that brings life to our environment,
wherever we are on this river.
May that water nurture us.

May we touch base with our sense of humor
and then flow freely with it.
May we find the journey on this river worth the effort.
May we find joy in all of us just being alive on the river.
May we endure the stress that this unrelenting change of
dementia brings.

Our prayer is for help to control what we can control,
our actions, our reactions, our attitudes.
We pray for help to stay afloat on this wild ride,
till she reaches her final shore.

RIDING THE RIVER

She never liked water,
being in it, or riding on it.
It's possible that she feared drowning.
Her younger brother fell through the ice
while skating on a pond and drowned.
She was watching him and couldn't save him.
Perhaps that is her fear of water,
even though she grew up near the shores of a river,
and later moved to a city on the same river.

Her fear, her dislike of the water
made her give us swimming lessons,
made certain we had life-saving skills.
We spent every Thursday after school at the Y,
taking swim class after swim class.
So we became accomplished swimmers
when we went to the Jersey shore.
She felt we were able to handle the ocean.
She couldn't come and get us if we were in trouble
in the water.

Now she is in trouble,
riding on the river of dementia.
All of our life-saving skills can't help her.
She's tossing and turning on that river,
sometimes finding a cove to shelter her,
but most times she's in the turbulent waves,
riding faster and faster.
At times she seems to go under,
and we can't reach her.
Those times we feel so helpless, so hopeless.

Sometimes we wish the ride to be over,
for her and for us.
Then a moment of clarity occurs.
We are astounded by her revelation,
but we know it's only for a moment.

Most moments are confusing,
awash with muddied thoughts and outpourings from her.
We want the river to clear her thoughts,
to wash away the unclear processes of her mind.
We know that's not possible.
The river can only take her where it wants to go.
And we are along for the ride,
riding together on the river of dementia.

WYOMING STYLE

While flying over this river of dementia,
I noticed how rugged the landscape was.
Wyoming is such a place of rugged beauty.
It is not a place for everyone,
but it is my place.

I think that living in Wyoming has prepared me
to travel on this river of dementia.
Living here has toughened my spirit.
Here you learn that you are not masters of everything
in your life.
The weather, the ruggedness of the landscape, the wind,
all condition you to go with the flow.
You can't fight the elements,
you learn to live with them,
and adjust yourself to the elemental reality.

Living in Wyoming gives me a slant on all that is
happening with my parents.
I try to adjust to their reality,
go with their flow.
Living in Wyoming teaches me to adapt, to bend, to revise,
to amend,
not to be caught up in one way of viewing things.
It teaches me to be open to the winds of change,
of chance, of other possibilities.
Living in Wyoming doesn't mean it is easier to deal with
my parents.

It just gives me a style on how I do.

FLYING OVER THE LARAMIE RIVER

I flew over the Laramie River,
seeing all the turns, swirls, eddies, and backwaters
from up above.
I watched the main course of the river turn back on itself,
form swirls and turns that led to dead ends,
backwaters with no outlet.

There was life there in those closed off channels.
Wildfowl came, antelope too,
to find a spot that was quiet,
in order to drink from the living waters.

Oh God, lead me beside the still waters,
so I can drink from your full cup,
so I can be filled again and go on,
traveling on the river of dementia.

CRAZY QUILT

"Scraps and pieces of fabric, sewn together with
embroidered threads in
various designs"

Life is like a crazy quilt.
We put our lives together, piece by piece, patch by patch.
A sunny yellow print,
a vibrant red stripe,
a soft square of blue,
an ominously dark black ribbon.
Colors flow, shapes emerge,
and a grand design evolves.
We add a baby flannel to a Parisian silk,
a beach bag print to a Sunday dress.

Sorrow joins our quilt,
and helps define the course of life.
It tones down the riotous, raucous patterns and colors,
colors of milestones reached and goals attained.

The silken threads tie it all together,
defining the borders, healing the ragged edges,
joining silk to corduroy,
satin to burlap,
velvet to cotton,
bringing beauty to all of it.
Oh the beautiful colors and designs!
What a quilt!
What a life well lived!

My Mother's memory is like a Crazy Quilt,
And she is forgetting piece by piece, scrap by scrap.

My Mother taught me how to sew.
"Save those scraps, they are good for something.
You never know when you'll need them,
for patching holes or mending tears."

There are so many holes in her memory now.
Where is the piece of fabric to patch the tears in her mind?
She remembers a fragment of memory here,
A piece there,
like a Crazy Quilt,
scraps and pieces,
some embroidered in colorful silks in stitched designs,
all put together to make a whole piece, a whole quilt,
a whole life.

Like my Mother.
Scraps of memories and experiences put together
to make a life.

We take scraps and visit them.
Sometimes it is a trip to her school days,
sometimes her marriage and first home,
sometimes to family long gone.
Scraps, a piece here, a piece there.

Like her conversation,
a piece here, a word there,
a mental photograph of yesterday.
Sometimes the memories come mumbled
and don't make sense.

Like pieces of a Crazy Quilt,
pieces don't seem to fit or blend or work together
when taken out of context.
But put the scraps, the pieces together,
add the silken threads of memory,
of a life well lived,
stitch the scraps together with cords of love,
a loving set of stitches, creating beauty,
a sharp dash of stitches showing movement,
a group of zig zag stitches showing excitement,
red stitches of anger,
black stitches of pain and sadness,
soft designs, harsh designs,
running stitches that connect the pieces,
and bring the story of pieces of life
into a whole lifetime,

a lifetime filled with joy, sadness,
pain, excitement,
anger, pride,
serenity, loss,
exhilaration, disappointment,
fulfillment.
A full quilt, a full life,
but not a finished life,
not yet.

So many pieces, so many stitches
pulled together to create this beautiful quilt
of my Mother's life.
What a magnificent life!

Pieces, scraps, threads.
like her memory now.
We pick up a piece, a scrap, and review it.
We take it, hold it in our hands,
review it, analyze it, agonize over it,
laugh over it, cry over it,
celebrate the joy it expresses,
share in the sadness it evokes.
Then we let it go –
and pick up another scrap at another time.

Sometimes she can't let it go.
That scrap of memory is painful.
The threads that connect it to the whole quilt
are torn and worn.
She picks at the threads,
trying to find the meaning to it all.
They are the bad memories, the sad times,
the unfilled times, the angry times.
She grieves over the scrap
as if it just happened.
We try to help her feel the pain,
validate her feelings and
help her to review it and accept it.

It's not easy –
She keeps picking at those threads.
I think maybe she'll pull out all the threads
that connect that scrap to the quilt –
then pull out the scrap
and throw it away.

She gets so angry at scraps of time
from the past.
She relives them again,
and burns with anger.
Sometimes it's directed at my Father,
sometimes at a lost relative,
sometimes at herself.

We visit her when she gets angry at long ago times.
We feel her pain with her.

We feel her tearing at the fabric.
We try to help her with closure.
We try to validate her feelings.
We try to help her move on.
We try to smooth the fabric of time.
We walk her to another scrap of memory,
one of joy, one of fulfillment.

Who knows what moment of time gone by,
what piece of fabric, what thread undone or torn
will hurt us and need to be reviewed and analyzed
and talked through before we let it go?
Maybe we need to review and analyze and talk through
those burned scraps of fabric,
those painful events in our own lives,
the painful threads that disconnect,
so we can feel them and then let them go,
and stand back and look at the quilt of our lives,
and say, like my Mom,
"It was beautiful, it is beautiful!"

"What a life!
Look how it all fit together!
Look at all the colors, all the patterns.

It needed every patch, every scrap.
Look at all the stitches that tied it together.
I wouldn't change a thing.
It's my life, my quilt.
It's my life well lived, well loved.
My beautiful Crazy Quilt!"

GOING CRAZY

I am slowly going crazy.
I hear them talking about me
everywhere I go.
Even my husband talks about me,
calls me names,
yells at me,
harps at me.

How am I going to live with this?
How am I going to handle this?
My daughter came over to visit.
I know she talks about me too.
They phoned my other daughter to do something.
DO SOMETHING!

Somebody do something.
How am I going to live like this?
I am going crazy.
Please, somebody help me.
Tell me I am not going crazy.
Make the bad times go away.
Make the bad thoughts go away.
Give me back to myself.
Give me back to my loved ones.
Give me back to my husband.
Give me back to my daughters.

Give ME back!

READING

I knew my mother's memory was slipping away
when she stopped sharing books with us.
Reading has been a great joy for all of us,
and books were always a great pleasure.
We used to exchange books amongst ourselves
as our own personal lending library.
"Take this and read it, you'll love it," she'd say.
We would spend long phone conversations
discussing plots and authors.

Now she cannot hold the thoughts long enough
to read a book.
"I still read," she tells me.
*"I look at the Reader's Digest.
I read every word in the newspaper,
sometimes two or three times to get the meaning."*

Now we are trying to 'read her,'
To discover what page she is on
so we can be on the same page.
How will this book end?

The story of her life –
a bit of Erma Bombeck and Betty Crocker,
a little of the Atlas and geography books,
a lot of the Bible and hymnals,
a pile of piano books and mystery novels,
crossword dictionaries and photo albums.

How will this book end?

LISTEN

Life is changing for Mom.
I live so far away that I feel helpless.
All I can do is give support, love, and listen.
That's the big thing
just to listen.

Listen to Mom when she tells me the same story
for the third time.
Listen when she complains about people, things, events.
Listen when she is forlorn about losing her memory.
Listen when she forgets the very special events of her life.
Listen when she forgets the very special events of my life.
Listen to her heart telling me she still loves me.
Listen to the message her loving hands tell me.
Listen to all the unspoken words of love shared with me.
Listen to the movements of her life
and how they gave me my being.
Listen to her love, pouring out to me in my memories.
Listen to the glorious being of love that she is.

Yes, I can listen - and hear the love.

ARE YOU LISTENING

*No one listens to me anymore.
They don't take the time to hear me.
They say I go on and on and on.
That's definitely wrong!
It's hard enough to get it out right the first time.*

*I try to tell them all what I'm thinking, what I'm doing.
All of them, my husband, my daughters.
Listen to me before I forget what I'm saying.
Hear what I am saying to you,
Listen with your inner ear.
Listen to my inner voice.
Hear my voice.*

Hear my pain.

TRIP TICS

This course of travel isn't in the approved AAA travel plan.
Mom and Dad belonged to AAA, and all our road trips were
planned out, page by page.
They would just turn the page to find the highway,
check out the area sights,
find a place to eat and a place to sleep.
Their life now has no road map,
no highway numbers to follow,
no known places to stop and visit,
no Trip Tic to follow,
no way to turn the page to see what will happen next.

What is happening next?
There is agony in not knowing.
There is the agony of traveling in uncharted territory.
We know where the destination is.
But how will we get there?
Who will show us the way?
Who will guide us along our journey?

We are in uncharted territory.
This is not the adventure we signed up for.
This is not on the road map.
How do we get off this road?
There are no exit ramps to other places.
There are no 'pull outs' along the road.
No rest areas.

But wait, I see some rest areas down the road.
There are times to take a breather,
times to recreate a memory of long ago,
times to dance in the moment,
times to dance together and reconnect.

And then we move on down that terrible road.
Will Dad be able to drive to the end?
Will he have a breakdown, physically or emotionally,
before it is over?

Will he be able to drive Mom to her final destination,
Or will he have to find an exit ramp first.

Where are those Trip Tics when you need them!

TRAVELING ON

What highway is this we're traveling on?
I don't remember being on this road before.
Are we lost?
Or am I the one who is lost?
Don't go so fast.
I can't keep up.

Everything is moving so fast, I can't keep up.
I don't recognize the road, the places on the side.
I don't recognize very much anymore.

Slow down - so I can think.
Slow down - give me time to remember.
Slow down - what's the hurry?
I don't know where we are.
I don't know where we're going.

But I think I know where we've been!

VACATIONS

The last two weeks of August were our vacation time.
We'd pack up and travel by car all over the East Coast
and mid-West.
Whatever we studied in history classes would be a good
choice for a trip.
Dad drove and Mom kept us occupied by singing, telling
stories, and playing games with us.
How lucky we were in the 1950s to travel
from Maine to Florida,
visit Washington, D.C. during the height
of the cherry blossoms,
see Mackinac Island and Wisconsin
and adventure through eastern Canada.
Mom would be the map reader
and the assistant navigator.
She kept us busy looking for places on the map.

It's hard to figure out where Mom is traveling now.
She has no road map, no travel guide,
no destination to look forward to.
She takes notes, writes down names and places.
We try to figure them out.
The scraps of paper are important to her.
They are her personal roadmaps.
Now the travels are the memories to her past.
We bring up a place and she recalls details of the trip.

We wish she could recall
the details of her latest activities.
Her memory now seems to go away on vacation.

I hope her trips are happy ones.

A FARAWAY PLACE

Mom and Dad loved to travel to see new places.
Growing up we traveled all over the USA.
Together Mom and Dad enjoyed trips
to Hawaii and Europe.
He tells the story of dancing with Mom
in the streets of Paris.
They've always loved to dance.

Now their trips are to a faraway place, not on any map.
Sometimes they both get lost.
We try to help them find their way.

But sometimes we get lost too.

PIANO

My mother taught herself how to play the piano
at fifty-two.
She could read music already,
and my sister taught her the rest.
Mom and Dad made sure we had piano lessons
growing up,
and bought us a superb instrument to play.
After we married and moved away,
Mom got with the program.

What fun she had playing the old favorites.
She'd call us and say, *"Listen to me play this song."*
How we marveled at her determination to learn.
My sister would give a lesson here and there,
and Mom learned them well.
Oh the joy she had sharing the music with Dad,
sharing with us, and achieving a personal goal.

When they moved from their Jersey home
they sold the piano.
Dad bought her a keyboard to use.
She played a little here and there.
Now her memory has lost those special skills.

We remember her playing her songs.

We remember the music.
We remember the music.

DO YOU HAVE THE TIME

Do you have the time?
Tell me the time.
Is it my time?
Is it our time?
Do you have the time?

I remember less and less.
I'm on a downhill slide.
How far will I go
before I don't remember me
and don't remember you?
Do you have the time?

Who is that stranger in the mirror?
Was that who I used to be
before I forgot to remember?
Do you remember?
Do you have the time?

I make lots of lists now,
names of places - of dates.
I remember the names,
but I forget why I made the list.
Do you remember?
Do you have the time?

Will I be remembered?
Will you remember me
when I forget?
Will someone remember me?
Who I am?
Who I was?
Do you have the time?

I was somebody once.
I was a good person,
a daughter,

a sister,
a wife,
a mother,
grandmother
great-grandmother.
I was a worker,
a volunteer,
a cook and baker,
a dancer.
Now that I remember,
how I love to dance.
Do you remember?
Do you have the time?

Help me remember.
I write the lists,
but forget where I put them.
I forget where I put lots of things.
Help me remember.
Will anyone remember me?
Will you remember?
Do you have the time?

Who am I?
Who did I used to be?
Who? Who?
Do you remember?
Do you have the time?

Do you know me.
who I used to be,
who I am?
If I don't know who I am,
how will I know what to do?
Will you help me?
Do you have the time?

How will I know the time?
How will I know the right time?
Do you have the time?

Will you help me?
Help me remember.
Help me when I'm frightened.
Help me when I get angry because I'm so scared.
Help me when I get so confused I cry.
Help me when I say or do something stupid.
Help me remember.
Help me be me.

Do you have the time?

MEMORIES

We need to cherish the memories of our mother.
Our memories are the best reality.
We can't face what we see now.
We retreat into the past,
just like her.

Are our memories all that is left of her?
The present reality is not real for her.
Not real for us either.

What is real anymore?

WHAT ARE THOSE LADIES SAYING ABOUT ME

What are those ladies saying about me?
I can tell they are talking about me.
It's the look on their faces.
They know.
They know I'm not all there.
I'm not here, I'm not there.
Where am I?
Where did I go?

I come and I go.
Sometimes I'm here,
and everything is good.
I know what I know.
I remember.

But there are other times, the bad times,
when I get confused, scared,
because I don't know what I'm doing,
what I'm supposed to do.
I forget names, people's faces.
They look like I should know them.
Do I know them?
Do they know me?

Do I know me?

FOR BETTER OR WORSE

I married you "for better or worse,
For richer or poorer.
In sickness and in health,
Till death do us part."
I promised to take care of you - until the end.
I never figured on it ending this way.
For over 66 years we've been together.
I promised to never leave you.
I will be with you always.

It scares me when you don't know me.
"You're not my husband," you yell.
I show you our wedding picture,
I show you our 50th anniversary portrait.
"That's not my husband," you cry.
I cry, too, deep inside, I cry.
How can you forget me, our time together?
For 66 years we've been together,
sharing everything.
Such joys we've had, such good memories.
We've had our poor days,
but most of the days have been rich days,
rich in love, rich in lives lived together.
We've raised two special daughters,
enjoyed grandchildren and great-grandchildren.
Oh, the years we've had together,
oh, the stories we can tell.
There have been some sad times, some tough times.
But we've come through them together,
became stronger –
Together.
We've shared everything –
Together.
We'll get through this –
Together.
I won't leave you.

Don't leave me.

DO YOU STILL LOVE ME

When I can't find the words,
when I can't find the thoughts,
when I can't find ME,
do you still love me,
when I am so confused, so mad?
Mad at you.
Mad at my memory.
Mad at myself.

Do you still love me?
When I accuse you of vile things,
when I am out of control,
when I can't calm down,
when I get so scared of losing all of me,
do you still love me?

Do you still love me?
When I am afraid of you
because I don't remember who you are?
do you still love me?

Yes I love you.
I will love you forever.
I will always love you.
I love you when you are my Mary, my joy.
I love you when we joke together.
I love you when we dance.
Oh, how I love you then.
I will love you forever.
Even when you forget,
even when you yell and scream at me,
even when you forget who I am.
I will love you forever.

I will never forget.

FOG

Mom's mind seems to grow more foggy.
Sometimes the fog lifts and she sees clearly the bright sun,
the colors of her present reality.
Sometimes the fog is soft and swirls around her,
teasing her with patches of memories.
Sometimes the fog is heavy and wet,
and dampens down any clear thought or reason.
Sometimes the fog is so dark we cannot see her at all,
and she cannot see us.

The fog will grow thicker and darker and
eventually swallow her up.
I hope for more days of sunshine to burn away the fog,
and time for all of us to be in the sunshine together.

THERE'S SOMEBODY HERE

*"I can't talk now
There's somebody here.
He's a neighbor,
come to visit me.
What's his name you ask?
I don't remember.
He comes around once in awhile for a visit.
Did you want to talk to him?
Here, let me introduce you to my daughter.
Hello - Who is this?
Who is this talking on the phone.
My daughter?
Who? What's your name?
Oh my name is Mary."*

"Mom, put Dad on the phone," I ask.
"Dad is not here right now," she tells me.
"I have a nice visitor watching TV with me."
"Mary, who are you talking to?" my Dad asks her.

"I don't know."

JUMBLE

Mom's mind is becoming like a jumble puzzle.
We try to figure out what the words mean,
what the sentences and stories mean.
Like a jumble puzzle, where you find the letters
to make a word,
but that is only half the discovery.
Now we have to figure out what the words mean.

My mother tells wonderful stories
and gives lots of information,
but we don't know the meaning.
We have the words, but don't get the gist of them.
Like a Jumble Puzzle,
lots of letters, lots of words,
But what do they mean?

What does she mean?

HIDING

"It's missing.
I can't find it.

I put it right there and now it's gone.
Did you take it and hide it from me?

How could you do that to me?
Why did you do that?

You know I need it.
Where did it go?

What am I looking for?"

DANCE WITH ME

"Dance with me, Mary."
My Dad asked Mom for the first dance,
and wound up being her partner for life.
They met at a dance,
and enjoyed 'the dance' for 68years.

I remember going to afternoon Tea Dances
and dancing with my Dad as a four year old.
My sister and I would watch our parents
jitterbugging in the kitchen to a special song.
And then Dad taught us how to dance.
'In the Mood' still triggers wonderful memories.

Mom and Dad continued the dance –
going to dinner dances, clubs, and parties.
Oh how they loved to dance.
Everyone would stop and watch them move.
My Dad was six feet tall and Mom a mere five feet two.
They danced like a dream, knowing each other's moves.
Now my Mom and Dad dance on Saturday night to
Lawrence Welk.
My sister and I enjoy watching them together,
seeing Dad lead and Mom following,
watching the love flow between the two of them,
like a river hugging the banks on both sides.

Mom and Dad continue the dance.
Sometimes dancing together is the trigger
that keeps my father in my mother's memories.
They still dance together.
I hope they will dance together for more dances.

The dance goes on, but the moves have changed.

FIND ME MY MEMORY

*"I feel so sad.
I feel so scared.
I can't remember names, people.
Will I forget you too?*

*Who is this man in my house?
Who are you?
You're not anyone I know!
I don't know you.*

*I am scared.
Tell me it's OK.
Tell me I'm not crazy.
Bring me back to me.
Make it all right again.*

Find me my memory."

TIME

The police came to my parent's home yesterday.
They came to investigate
a possible domestic violence scene.
Some neighbor called them after finding my mother
screaming in the parking lot.
"Help me, he's trying to kill me," she yelled,
as my father tried to bring her back into the apartment.
"Let me go, don't touch me, who are you?" she screamed.

"I'm your husband, John," my father told her.
She didn't believe him.

And then he told the police about her condition,
showed them the letter from her doctor,
told them about her hallucinations.
They understood.
She didn't.

She was agitated and wouldn't go with him
into the apartment.
Some neighbors tried to calm her and she came around.
It takes time.
My dad has the time.

He has the love that conquers time.

MISS YOU

Oh, Mom, I miss you.
I miss your caring words, your loving touch.
I miss your special ways of loving me.
How much longer before you go away for good?

"For good"
- what an odd way to explain you are gone forever.
Will it be "for good"
when you can't remember any of us anymore?
Will it be "for good"
when you are free of painful memories?
Will it be "for good"
when you only live moments of past days?
Will I still be your daughter
when your mind is gone "for good?"

You'll always be my mother "for good."

BAKING

I now have my Mother's and Grandmother's wood pastry
board.
Mom doesn't bake anymore.
She doesn't create those delicious pastries I remember
from my childhood.
My sister and I knelt on chairs, next to her
as she created rich goodies.
We learned how to make the dough,
turn it out on the board,
pat it and roll it and roll it again.
Add the nut and fruit fillings, then cut and bake them.
We'd wait, a watchful waiting at the oven door,
watching the Kifli and the Kolach,
the Hungarian pastries, bake.
Only Mom knew when they were done, when they were
ready.

When I use the board, I remember her hands
kneading and rolling.
I feel her hands on mine,
adding a touch of flour to make the dough less sticky.
I see my Grandmother looking over my shoulder
as I create the pastry,
Nodding her head and saying in Hungarian, 'jol,' good.
I see my Mother sitting across the table from me,
watching me,
still guiding me, guiding my hands.

The simple task of kneading and rolling
brings tears to my eyes,
and makes the dough sticky.
I add more flour, a pinch here, a pinch there.
Will I be able to add 'flour' to the sticky dough
of her present reality?
Will I be able to help my father and my sister
roll out the dough?

I watch my father and sister pat and
roll the dough together,
working as a team now that my mother
is no longer the pastry chef.
My father and sister continue the tradition.
I feel separate, not a part of the scene.
They are the ones who must make the pastry now.
They are the ones in her present reality.
I am too far away to bake with them.
I try to bring 'recipes' to them,
'How To' guides to help them figure out
how to care for Mom.
I have quite a collection in my cookbook.

I hope they try the new ones.
The old ones don't work anymore.

NO MORE BAKING

I gave my daughter my wooden pastry board.
I don't use it anymore.
Arthritis in my hands causes me too much pain
to use the rolling pin.
The arthritis in my mind causes me
to forget the recipes anyway.
She will use it well.
Just like me before her and my mother before me.

All the memories of flour, sugar, eggs, spices,
and nuts are in that board.
How we loved to bake and create Hungarian pastries.
Now it's my daughter's turn to bake and grind the nuts.
She will use it well.
I will miss it,
I will miss it.

Now I am one of the nuts.

SHE LOST HER MEMORY

*I lost my memory.
I don't know where it went.
I keep looking for it here and there.
Is it in the pile of papers on the table?
Maybe it's in this bunch of old letters.
Are they old letters or did we just get them?
Get what?
What did you ask?*

*Oh, letters, yes letters.
Did you write me a letter?
It must be here in this pile.
What was I looking for?
Oh, papers and papers.
I need to organize them.
They belong in this box.
Where did I put them?
Where do they go?*

*Let me clean up this mess.
Should I throw them away?
I'll put these away.
Now, where do they go?
Ah, here's a spot in the closet.
I'll just put them here.
Why am I in this closet?
What am I looking for?*

*Where is my memory?
Where did it go?*

MY SISTER

My sister is the one who has the burden
of caring for our parents.
She is the first to be called,
the first to come over and help them.
She has such a tough task to handle.
She never knows what will be happening
when Dad calls in the middle of the night.
She never knows if Mom will be angry,
scared, or just a little upset.
But she goes,
and she gives,
and she is there.

She takes a deep breath and goes to them.
Dad can depend on her.
Mom can depend on her.
I can depend on her.

Who can depend on me?
I am not there.
My sister and Dad have the burden.
I am not there.

But I care.
I care for all of them.
Even if I am not there.

Even when my heart is breaking
Because I am not there.

SISTER IS UP CLOSE AND PERSONAL

I wanted my Mom and Dad near me
so I could enjoy their company,
share in their lives, at this twilight time.
I never expected this.
My sister tried to explain what was happening,
what would be happening next.
I really didn't believe it.
I couldn't get a handle on this.
Dad is slowing dying and Mom is going crazy.
That's to put it bluntly.

I'm the one who is here.
I am the one they turn to call,
in the middle of the night,
while I am at work,
when I'm out with my husband and friends,
when I need down time and time to be alone.
I'm the one to take them to the doctor, their dentists,
their specialists.
Me - Me - Me.

I don't know if I can handle this.
My sister tells me to join a Support Group.
Yah! When do I have the time!
She sends me reams of information about Mom's disease,
But I don't want to read it.
I don't want to know what could happen next.
I don't want to know.
I want my Mom and Dad.
I want them as they were, my Mommy and Daddy.
I don't like the changes.
I don't want them to die.
Not yet, not like this.

My sister comes and visits.
She tries to help,
sends me info to read,
sends me goodies to enjoy.
I wish she could send me HER.
Take my place for awhile.
Give me a break.
I didn't sign up for this ending.

Or did I?

AT A DISTANCE

Here I am 2,000 miles away,
at a distance,
wishing I could be there to help more.
Sometimes I feel so useless.
Yes, I know a lot about dementia.
After all, it's my profession.
But these are my parents,
this is my sister,
and I am here,
at a distance.

I try to give information,
listen to the calls of desperation and pain,
from my father, my sister, and my mother.
I can't change things.
I can't make it better.
I am here, at a distance.

I'm dealing with disease and breakdown, too.
Between my spouse and me, we're dealing with cancer.
But the breakdown seems to grab me emotionally.
Some days I feel so drained.
I want to do so much for them all.
I visit and help when I'm there.
I fill up with love from all of them.
Love to sustain me until I get the calls again.

When I feel the pain again.

At a distance.

TIDBITS

Laughter now hides in strange places.
Like finding a box of tissues in the freezer.
*"That's in case I need them for later.
I know they're in there."*

Pieces of paper are all over the place.
*"That's in case I need to remember something.
I write it down, but I forget why I wrote it.
At least I can still write!"*

Or finding photos all over her house.
"I am trying to remember those people."
I find photos of our family, my children, their trips,
scattered, like her mind.
"Leave them out, they help me remember the old days."

My Mother loves her onion rings and we get them often.
She says, *"I love onions. Onion is my middle name."*
Her middle initial is O for her maiden name.

I worry about my future and how I will live
on a reduced income.
She tells me, *"It's not what you've earned that matters,
it's what you've learned."*

She tells me not to wait until retirement to live my life
because what you wait for may not come.
Live today and enjoy today.
Do the things you plan on doing when you retire - NOW.
Travel, dance, read, play, enjoy - NOW.

"This is your mother telling you this, so listen up!"

DOWNSIZING STUFF

When I last visited my parent's apartment,
we downsized.
My sister and I packed up and put away
the china, silver, and crystal.
We sorted through items from their home,
from our home.
We sorted through memories.
"Remember this," we'd say to each other,
going through knick knacks and stuff.
They haven't died.

But there we were,
sorting out, dividing up our childhood,
our parents lives.
There they were,
watching us, giving direction.
What were they thinking as we handled
the everyday stuff
of their lives?
Packing up the 'good stuff' was like saying,
they are done with those things.
And they are, they are.

My heart was breaking as I packed up
the silver tea set.
Tears fell as I wrapped dishes and glasses.
The old familiar pieces became
my pieces, my sister's pieces.
We packed up pieces of our parents lives.
Now our pieces.

That's how we remember.
We pick up a piece, touch it, remember.
Like pieces of a crazy quilt,
a piece here, a piece there,.
all sewn together to make a life.
My pieces, her pieces, their pieces,
now our pieces.

It's not over.
It's just moving into another dimension,
another direction.
And so are we all,

So are we all.

NOT DONE

They are not done with living.
The next step is Assisted Living.
Another loss in their travels on the river.
More dependent on others now.
They need more than we can provide.

This journey is not over,
but it's moving faster.
It's another step in the loss of identity.
It's another form of downsizing.

It's another form of goodbye.

STUFF

They're going through my stuff.
I don't like this.
It's my stuff.
It doesn't matter that I don't use it.
It's still my stuff.
I like touching the Lenox,
Running my fingers over the glasses.

I remember.
I remember.

MY SEWING MACHINE

Don't take that away.
I may need it yet.
What will I do if I tear a hem?
I need the machine to fix it.
It's my sewing machine.
I've always had it.
Don't take it away.
It's mine.

I don't remember how to get it started.
Like me, sometimes,
I don't remember how to get me started.
Don't take it away.
It's mine.

I need to hold on to it.
I need to hold on to my mind.
I may need it to mend the tears there, too.

Don't take it away.
It's all I have left to fix things.
Don't take it away.

Don't take me away.

SEWING MACHINE

My Dad asked us to take the sewing machine away.
Mom doesn't need it anymore.
They moved it from their New Jersey home
to their Carolina apartment.
It was a part of their home, their life, their past.
It came with them.
Now it needs to go.

I remember Mom making me a taffeta skirt.
It was for a special tea party in junior high.
She took the lining out of an old coat and
made a beautiful full skirt for me.
Whether she sewed or just mended,
the Singer sewing machine was a part of our lives.

I learned how to sew on that machine, too.
I wasn't interested much at that time,
but I learned.
Mom taught me.
She even taught Dad how to use the machine.

Mom's Grandmother was a seamstress,
And Mom wore beautiful dresses.
Her Mother, my Grandmother, had a treadle machine
that we enjoyed playing with.
Mom learned how to sew on that oldie.
Her sewing abilities got her a job
at a handkerchief factory in her youth.

She sewed beautiful things for her two daughters.
For special outfits, Mom would have our outfits
made by a dressmaker.
When she didn't have enough time she found Nelly.
My sister and I would wear matching suits and dresses.
The dressmaker would do the designing
and some of the sewing,
and then Mom would do the rest.

We looked special because we wore unique outfits.
Mom wanted us to look classy.
And we did.
Just like our classy Mom.

Now the sewing machine isn't used anymore.
It's looking for a new home,
like Mom.
She's looking for a new home, too.
We're waiting for an assisted living apartment.
for her care and Dad's too

It's time.
Time for them to be waited on and looked after.
Time for them to have meals provided and rooms cleaned.
Time for them to get help when they need it.
Time for them to have help
when they don't think they need it.
Time to look for a new home.
Time to give up the old.

Time to say they need help.
Time to find it for them.
Time to let go.

Time to take the sewing machine away.

INCONTINENCE

My mother is incontinent.
Dad called to let me know she cannot control her bladder.
She either dribbles constantly or gushes and flows.
We have to use incontinence products, diapers,
to hold in the flow.
We never know when her urine will overflow
And stain and ruin her clothing.

It's like that with her thoughts now, too.
She is incontinent of thoughts and reason and words.
We never know what will flow out of her mouth,
what thoughts she will try to put into words,
what words she will try to put into sentences
to tell us her thoughts.

Sometimes she dribbles - words, thoughts.
Sometimes she gushes with a story of long ago events ,
made up events that have no history, no meaning.
Just a hodge-podge of thoughts and feelings.

There are no incontinent products to hold in the flow.
There are no products to help clean the stain
of her hurtful words.
There are no products to mend the pain my father feels
when she doesn't know him as the love of her life.

But my father's love overflows and knows no boundaries.

It will never be dry.

LOST CONTROL

I cannot hold my water..
I used to dribble a bit,
or just barely get to the bathroom.
Now I can't wait anymore.
It comes when it comes.

I've lost control,
control over my body now, too.
I know I've lost control over my mind.
I see it in my family's faces when I am not 'all there.'
I don't know where I am anymore.

I don't like it here.

DRESSING UP

Mom always dressed up for the occasion.
What a classy lady!
She expected her daughters to be dressed up
and look classy, too.
Hats and gloves for church,
Dresses when we visited her at the bank.

Now she forgets to wear her undergarments,
and her pants are stained from her incontinence.
She has to wear adult diapers.
No way is that a classy look!

Sometimes the combinations of her outfits are a little odd,
so we put outfits together on a hanger for her.
My sister will put clothing out the night
before an occasion,
but Mom still picks her own.

It's hard to redirect her.
"I'm so humiliated that you think I don't know
how to dress," she says
as we try to adjust an outfit.
She looks sad and then gets mad
at losing her sense of autonomy,
at losing the choice to pick her own clothing.

This was the lady who raised us to be ladies.
Now we are assisting this person
to look presentable in public.
Dad loves her so much he doesn't want
to argue with her about her choices,
so he accepts whatever she chooses.
Sometimes, she looks a bit jumbled up.

It's hard to see this lady, this classy woman,
looking like a bag lady.

ALL DRESSED UP

I know how to dress up.
Leave me alone and let me pick my own clothes out.
Why are you telling me what to do!
Don't you think I can do this by myself!
I've been dressing myself for 90 years now.
I know what I want!

Or do I?

I can't find the pants that go with this top.
Where did I put them?
Oh, here they are in the bathroom.
Who put these over the shower curtain rod!
Why aren't they in my closet!
Who moved them!
Why are they a little damp!
I'll just put these on.
They'll dry soon.
Now I'm ready to go.

What do you mean I can't wear these pants!
They are a set, they go together.
So what if they are a little wet.
No, I did not wet them myself.
They just got a little wet.
I can still wear them.
Don't tell me what to wear.
I know what I'm doing.

Don't I?

COOKING

How my mother loved to cook and bake.
Oh, the delicious cooking aromas
that drifted out the door
when I returned from school!
Pot roast, chicken soup, beef stew, chicken paprikas,
all took time to prepare and slow cook
to bring to its perfect end,
all the ingredients needed, all the spices to make it tasty.
And she rarely used a cook book to make it happen.

Caring for my mother now is like preparing
a slow cooked meal.
It takes time to prepare her to go out,
whether shopping, church, or to go out to dinner.
Time to get her ready, to talk her through the process.
Time to direct and redirect and redirect her again.
Time to gather all the things she needs.
Time to get the ingredients, the clothes, the
undergarments together.
Time to gather them and assist her.
Time to make her presentable, to make her
ready to go public.

It takes time and energy to create this stew pot.
There are no recipes to care for her.
We are in new territory.

We need a cook book now.

THE COOK IS DONE

*I forgot to add the sour cream to the goulash last week.
What a dummy I've turned out to be.
I goofed and put Cool Whip topping in it instead.
What a yucky mess that turned out to be!
Thank goodness my daughter caught it.
What's the matter with me?
I can't remember the simplest recipes anymore.*

*They won't let me cook anymore.
I put the plastic container in the oven to cook.
We threw that mess away, too.
What used to be second nature to me is gone.
Now I don't know what to do.
Thank goodness I taught my husband how to cook.
He does ok, too.
But not me.
I'm not ok.*

*What used to bring me joy now causes me great worry.
I don't trust myself.
I don't trust me.*

*Will they forgive me?
This cook is done!*

STARVING

"I'm starving," my mother said.
"That stingy man wouldn't give me anything to eat."

She points to my father and berates him
after he has prepared three pancakes,
eggs, and sausage for her.
He tries to get her to eat,
but she refuses his offering of food.
He tries to orient her to reality and to his love,
but she refuses his offering.
He's the one starving here.

She's refusing him more and more lately.
Dad used to bring her around emotionally,
but that is getting more and more difficult.

She stays away for longer periods.
My sister has to intervene more and more.
Mom keeps talking about *"that man."*

That man loves her to pieces.

Now he's falling into pieces.

MORE CALCIUM

Growing up we learned our table manners early.
Going out to dinner was a treat.
We were expected to be on our best behavior.
We learned how to order from a menu,
and were expected to behave appropriately at the table.

Mom still enjoys eating out,
but the rules have changed.
We order for her, as there are
too many choices and they confuse her.
She seems to eat the oddest combinations.
Any condiments on the table might end up
as an additive to her plate.

She always has a reason for her unusual behaviors.
While eating at a restaurant
she took several coffee creamers
and slathered them over her chicken entree.
We tell her it's creamer for her coffee.
She tell us,
"You always say I need to eat more calcium!"

LIFESAVERS

Mom loved Lifesaver candies.
She doled them out to us one at a time
when we went to the Saturday matinee movies.
My sister and I would dicker over the flavors.
"You got the last coconut, the next one's mine."
Mom enjoyed passing out the candies.
She was always our lifesaver.
Who will be her lifesaver?

She was always there for us.
Whenever we felt a hole in our lives,
she found a life saver to save us.
Now who can save her?
Who can listen and understand her now?
Who will fill the holes in her mind?
Who will be her lifesaver?

I think there are only lemons left in that roll.

SWIMMING

We grew up spending summers down at the shore.
We weren't allowed to go in deep water
until we knew how to swim.
So during fall, winter, and spring we took swimming
lessons at the local Y.
Every Thursday we trooped over to the Y
with Mom accompanying us.
She sat in the bleachers watching us learn how to float and
then swim.
My sister and I loved the water,
so Mom kept giving us lessons.
Swimming, advanced swimming, diving, water ballet,
Junior lifesaving,
anything to be in the water.

In the summers we would pack a small suitcase
with our bathing suit, cap and towel,
and go to the city pool.
It was twenty city blocks away, quite a hike.
We would walk the 7-8 blocks to Livingston Avenue
and wait for the bus to take us the rest of the way.
Sometimes we would just keep walking,
and when the bus came,
we ignored it because we were close enough.
Mom didn't drive so we walked everywhere
or took a city bus.
We would have an afternoon playing in the pool,
and then ride the bus back home.

Weekends we went down to the shore with Mom and Dad.
We couldn't wait to be in the water.
It would be freezing cold, but we got acclimated
and spent most of our time riding the breakers.
Mom would stand on the shore, at the edge of the water
watching us closely,
always knowing where we were.
I drove her nuts because

I loved to be under the waves and swimming underwater.
Mom couldn't swim and had a fear of the water,
Yet she made sure we had plenty of time in the water,
and the lessons to know what to do.

We are trying to figure out what to do about Mom.
She keeps plunging into the water
and we know she can't swim.
We are her lifesavers,
but we don't know where the shore is.
So we are hanging on,
hanging on to her and to each other.

Sometimes all you can do is tread water.

MEMORIES

We need to cherish the memories of our Mother.
Our memories are the best reality.
We can't face what we see now.
We retreat into her past,
just like her.

Are our memories all that is left of her?
The present reality is not real for her.
Not real for us either.

What is real anymore?

CHURCH

We lived around the corner from our church,
So every Sunday we walked to the services,
Sunday school first, church next,
and then visiting time,
catching up with friends,
showing off our latest outfits,
planning our Sunday afternoons.

As the Hungarian people in our
urban neighborhood moved to the suburbs,
and the church membership declined,
Mom and Dad continued to be faithful leaders.
They never missed a Sunday service,
and gave so much of themselves to the church.
This place was my father's boyhood sanctuary,
and then later my family's place of worship.

Moving away from their home was also
moving away from a church family.
There is a long history there.
Now my parents attend a church near their new place.
They are the oldest members at that parish,
and receive recognition for their constancy
and devotion to God.

When I visit, we attend services together.
Mom finds the pages of the hymns and readings,
but she doesn't sing anymore.
She smiles sweetly at me as I sing the hymns,
and turns the pages to find her place for the
next part of the service.

It brings me joy to hear her say the Lord's Prayer and
Apostle's Creed.

Some things are never forgotten.
I hope she knows that God has not forgotten her,
and there is sanctuary here.

Is there any sanctuary for us?

GOD AND ME

Okay, God, why are you doing this to me?
Why are you making me go crazy?
What did I do to deserve this?

They all think I am crazy.
I think I am crazy.
Do you think I am crazy?

I think about you a lot, God.
I wonder when you will call me home.
All my loved ones are there with you now.

This man says he is my special loved one.
But I don't know him.
Do you know him?
Should I know him?

Should I love him?
Should I love you?

LONELY

Have you ever been lonely?
Have you ever been blue?
Have you ever loved someone
just as I love you?

Mom sang that song to my sister and me as a lullaby.
She wasn't great at singing.
Somehow this popular song became our goodnight song.

Now it is Dad's goodnight song.
I see my Dad in these words,
Feeling lonely and blue as his beloved wife disappears
into the waters of dementia.

Loving her and losing her.
His goodnight song to her.

LONELINESS

I am so lonely.
Is there anyone who cares?
Help me.
It hurts and hurts.
I don't know where it aches.
It just does.

Don't give me another pill.
I've had plenty already.
I don't want anymore.
Leave me alone.

No!
Don't go!
Don't go.
I am so lonely.

Does anyone care?

HOME AGAIN

She wants to go home again.
Dad thinks she's sad about leaving
their home in New Jersey.
That's not where she wants to go.
She's confused and wants to go home to a place
where she remembers,
a place where she feels safe,
a place where she knows the people.
I tell Dad she feels like she's in a foreign country.
She doesn't recognize the furniture,
she doesn't recognize him or us.
Going home isn't to a place anymore.
It's to another solar system.

"Dad," I say, "Imagine waking up in China
in a strange room.
Some strange person is telling you what to eat,
what to wear.
That person is telling you to go to bed with him.
Think about how frightened you would be."

That's where Mom is,
In a foreign country now.
And we can't go there with her.

We can't get through customs.

HOME

I want to go home.
Please take me there.
I am afraid.
I don't know who you are.
Do you know who I am?

Take me home.
Make me safe.
I don't know this place.
I am afraid.

I pretend I know you.
But you scare me.
All of you scare me.
Take me home.

Please, hurry me home.
Find my place.

I can't find myself anymore.

SLIP SLIDING AWAY

How far will she go?

She's slip sliding away.
She's drifting away.

How far will she go?

THE BUS

We always took the Number 4 or Number 6 bus
to visit our Grandmom.
Mom walked us downtown so we could catch the bus.
Sometimes we would pack a small suitcase with our pj's
and a change of clothes.
Sometimes it was just for a late afternoon of fun,
dinner, and a visit.
Dad would come and pick us up in the evening
and home we'd go.
Sometimes we'd spend the night
and he'd get us the next day.

It was always a fun time to visit our country grandparents.
Grandmom made chocolate pudding for every visit,
and would have it cooling on the porch when we arrived.
It became our welcome mat.

Now we are trying to figure out
what bus to take to Mom's place.
We don't know where the bus stop is.
It's hard to figure out if she is there for an afternoon,
or whether she will be there for the next few days.

Who will pick her up and take her home?
Will Dad be able to find her?
Will she be able to find Dad?
Will she remember he is her welcome mat?

He will always be her welcome mat.

MOTHER LOVE

We love you for being the best Mother a daughter
could ever have.
For being a role model for us,
for showing us what a loving woman is all about,
forgiving all the crummy stuff we pulled while growing up,
for teaching us how to cook, bake, and,
yes, even how to clean.

We love you for showing us how to dress and shop,
and how to look and act like a classy lady,
for giving us the wonderful world of books,
for doing all those fun things with us,
for walking with us everywhere.

We love you for all the times you just sat and listened,
for leading us by example and showing us the way,
for your faith in God and your faith in us,
for trusting in God's guidance, when perplexed with us,
for loving us no matter what.

We love you for all the sacrificing you did
to see that we got what we needed,
for never giving up when things got tough,
for working hard helping Dad with the business
while working yourself,
and still cooking up a storm at home.

We love you for helping us when times got tough,
for always believing in us,
that we could do anything we put our minds to,
for loving unconditionally.

You have lived a wonderful, loving, giving life.
Now let us help you find peace and strength to deal with
the rest of your life.

What an honor to have a Mother like you to love.

We love you unconditionally.

PRISONER

"Why are you keeping me a prisoner?"
She asks my father as her tries to keep her from escaping.
"Let me go outside, I want to go away."

He knows and he wants to protect her.
Protect her from her memory loss,
Protect her from herself.
She doesn't get it.
And neither does he.

Neither one can escape.

EYES

My Mother lost her left eye to cancer while in her thirties.
She's written up in the New England Journal of Medicine.
She survived a new procedure.

How did she do it?
She survived and thrived, in spite of it.
Those days, there were no support groups,
no one to help one "get through it."
She did it alone.
But not quite alone.
She had love and support from my Father,
and love and support from her family.

She adjusted to a different world view.
Wearing a black eye patch was not for her.
As soon as she could she got a prosthesis
to help her to look more normal.
She couldn't see out of her left eye,
But she could see the world from her right.
She never became dependent on someone to drive her,
to take her places.
She walked and we walked with her.
She rode the bus and we rode with her.

The only thing we noticed as children was
she never filled our glasses up high enough for us.
I never noticed she was sightless in one eye.
She was a dynamo - nothing slowed her down.

When she retired from her banking job,
she volunteered for Prevention Blindness.
It was another full-time "job" for her.
She was there for others who lost vision in an eye.
"You have another eye," she would say,
"You still can see."

She never felt diminished by it.
I think it empowered her,
to speak up for others,
to speak up for herself.

My daughter shares the same shade of gray in her eyes.
And she shares the spirit of surviving.
I remember walking with my Mother through busy streets.
I would start out walking on her left side,
and she would say *"Walk on my right side so I can see you,
You don't have to protect me."*
No we didn't have to protect her then.

Now we all have to protect her.
She can't walk these streets alone.
We don't know what will be coming from
the left or right side anymore.
We don't know if there is a right side anymore.
We don't know how she will react to anything.

These streets are unknown and scary.
This city is unknown and scary.
We see the river threading its way through the cityscape.
We get directions from the river.
We see movement.
We see the river caressing the banks,
or storming against the shore.
Like my Mother.

We see the Raritan River of her youth, of her city life,
flowing to the ocean, the sea.
Now the river goes by another name.
But it flows to the same ocean, the same sea.

We're flowing on it together.

FORK IN THE RIVER

Our journey has taken a new fork on the river.
Mom finds her own watercourse, her own channel.
We try to float along with her.
Sometimes we drift in the shallows,
sometimes we cling to her in the rushing water.

What will happen when the floodtide comes?
What will be left of us?
What will be left of her?

Will we all be washed clean,
or muddied and sullied by our emotions,
our own needs and wants?

RUST

*"I can't stay long.
My cousin had a baby and I have to help her."*
Her cousin died 6 months ago at the age of 90.
Mom is remembering events of the past,
trying to connect them to her present reality.

Births and deaths seem to be etched in our memories.
It doesn't matter when they occurred -
those memories stay.
The joys remain, the pain remains.

The memory rusts away.

GOODBYE

When will I say my last goodbye to my Mother?
How soon will my Mother not know me?
When will she not recognize me?
There are times when she asks,
"Who is that woman in the kitchen?"
I tell her I am her daughter.
I see the lost look in her eyes.
She doesn't know me.
But she fakes it well.

If I am lucky,
She comes around and recognizes me.
She hugs me and smiles.
I am her daughter again.
I hope to be her daughter for a long time yet.
It doesn't matter if I am a part-time daughter.

She will always be my full-time Mother.

A LITTLE BIT OF DYING

*"I'm down in the dumps here.
We're getting ready for a funeral."*

"Who died, Mom?" "Whose funeral is it?" I ask.
"MINE,"
"It's my funeral" she tells me.

She dies a little every day.
A piece of her memory shrivels up and is torn from the
fabric of her quilt.
We try to stitch it back with a bit of reality.
But that doesn't work very well any more.

Now we go to another patch and reminiscence.
That seems to work better.
It's hard to let those memories go.
It's even harder to know she can't retrieve them anymore.

She's lost on the river.
Those memories drowned in the whirlpool
that was once her mind.
How much longer can we hold on to her,
before she's pulled into the vortex and drowns?

WATER

It's raining now.
Sometimes it's a drizzle, sometimes a downpour.
But it's definitely raining.

During a recent trip, we were visited by a deluge,
and the apartment parking lot became flooded.
Dad strode to the car, getting soaked in the process.
Mom and I skirted the water and waded
through to the other side.

Dad continues to get soaked, diving into her reality.
Sometimes he doesn't have enough time to dry out before
the next storm hits.
Mom still can wade through and get to the other side.
But she gets confused
because she has to take a different path.

The paths of her old days were deluged with rain and
followed by sunshine.
Now we find more rain.
It's definitely raining.

Mom has never liked the water.
She always preferred to stand at its edge.
But she needs the water –
washing, bathing, eating, drinking.

Does she remember the water of her mother's womb?
Does she remember the water of her baptism?
Does she remember the waters of her daughters' births?

She would quote a favorite poem to me as a child,
"The Rhyme of the Ancient Mariner."
It dealt with water, too.
"Water, water everywhere, and all the boards did shrink.
Water, water everywhere nor any drop to drink."

Now her mind is shrinking,
And she has difficulty taking any water to drink.
We encourage her to drink, to be hydrated,
but she doesn't comply.
"I drink plenty," she says as she sips a bit here and there.

It's not enough for her system.
She becomes dehydrated,
and then the behaviors start.
She gets cranky and ornery.

Even though it's raining on her parade,
it's not enough water.
It's like she's dried out and her memory begins to shrink.

Just like the Ancient Mariner.

FLOATING AWAY

*They're always making me drink.
I take a sip of water, but I'm not thirsty.
I drink plenty.
I had a cup of tea for breakfast, didn't I?*

*I love my tea!
Don't forget my lemon!
Is that another glass of water?
That's too much.
I'll have to go again.*

*Don't make me drink anymore.
I'm too full of water.
I'll float away.*

*I'm floating away as it is.
I don't want to float away forever.
I can't help it anymore.*

There I go.

FLOWING, FLOATING, OR DROWNING

How do we flow on this river of life?
We're not in the shallows anymore.
We're in deep water.
So far, we crest the waves that Mom throws our way.
We're not drowning.
She's not drowning,
Not yet.

We're holding our heads up.
Sometimes she goes under and we can't find her.
It takes a while, but we can bring her back to shore.
How long before we are caught in the current of her
dementia,
and can't bring her back to dry land?

It's a different shore we're looking at now.

TEA

How my mother loved a cup of tea,
good old Lipton tea bags with a slice of lemon.
My sister and I would enjoy sharing a cup of tea with her,
sitting at the kitchen table.
Sometimes we used the tea pot and
brewed a pot for all of us.
Then it was a real tea party.
How that connected the three of us.

Dad is a coffee drinker.
We'd share a cup of coffee with him, too.
We had more milk than coffee in our cups.
Tea was our ladies special brew.

I only drink tea now,
just like my mother had it, with a twist of lemon.
Only I add a touch of honey to mine.
Mom was like a touch of honey, with a sweet nature.
But watch out for the sharpness of the lemon!

I now have Mom's silver tea service.
It brings back memories of tea parties from long ago,
of having company and using the good china,
eating in the dining room.

Every time I use the tea pot I honor my mother.
I honor the memories of childhood tea parties
and grown-up parties.
I honor my mother's joy of having people over,
of preparing a dinner feast or a dessert.
I honor her ability 'to do it up and do it right.'

I honor the tradition of serving others
through the serving of food and drink,
through the serving of tea and coffee,
through the serving of herself to my father,
my sister and me,

through the serving of her special gifts to her church and
community.

It was her tea service,
now it is mine.
It's my turn to pour and serve.
Her hands are on mine as I lift the heavy silver pot.

Now it's my turn to pour.
Now it's my turn to serve.

SWEETNESS

My Mother was such a sweet lady.
I don't see much of that anymore.
Now her voice crackles with irritation, with angst.
She has lost her sense of direction.
How she loved hot tea with lemon and sugar.
Now I only see the lemons in her life.

What happened to the sweetness?

MEDS

Mom's meds aren't working well.
The behavior drug doesn't seem to be effective anymore.
We need to do something else.
Her doctor has prescribed a drug holiday,
So Mom will enter a Psych unit of a hospital.
Ten days to evaluate her and review her meds.
Ten days of respite time for Dad.
Maybe he'll get to sleep through the night,
to be ready for the next battle.

Their interactions have turned into battles.
What was a loving, giving relationship,
a marriage based on trust and understanding,
has turned into a bloody battlefield of the mind.

She accuses him of trying to kill her, of starving her,
of keeping her under his guard.

He quietly weeps inside
as she throws accusations at him,
hurls epithets at him,
directs her rage at him.

He weeps.

So does she.

CAN HE STILL DO IT

Mom is in the hospital going through a drug review.
Her behaviors have been off the wall for a while.
This step was important to help us figure out
why her behavior is "out there."

My Dad is home alone for the day.
He finally gets to sleep.
He visits for an hour and a half each evening,
and sees the progression of her disease.
Does he really see how far she's gone?
He still wants to take her home and care for her.
Can he meet her needs?

I don't think so!

Can he stop her from leaving the apartment
and wandering off?
I don't think so!

Can he give her the meds she needs, when she
needs to take them?
I don't think so!

Can he keep her hydrated and feed her?
I don't think so!

Can he keep her oriented to her present reality?
I don't think so!

Her exiting seeking behavior still exists.
How can he keep her safe?
She doesn't remember him
when it's time to take her meds.
How will he give them to her then?
She doesn't remember who he is when he cooks for her.
How will he keep her nourished?

She doesn't remember him and
wants to get away from him.
She doesn't want to sleep in the same bed.
"I'm a married woman, I don't sleep around," she says.
Is he still able to take care of her?
I don't think so!

His love has nourished her for over 68 years.
It's not enough anymore.
She needs a different kind of caregiving now.

I think so!

ENERGIZER BUNNY

Mom is constantly talking.
She goes on and on and on.
We can't figure out the whys.
She's telling a good story,
but we can't figure out who the characters are,
what they are doing,
and what's the relationship with her.
On and on and on she goes

like an energizer bunny.

ON THE MOVE

She's a woman on the move.
On and on and on she goes.
Where she'll stop nobody knows.
"I want to go home," she states.
It's not any place we know about.
Perhaps it's going home to a memory place,
a memory of her childhood
where her mother and father lived.
a time when she knew they would take care of her
and keep her from all the unknowns.

It's all unknown now.
She can't touch base with much it seems.
Her home, her space with Dad is unknown to her.
Her daughter's home is another unknown.
Sometimes her daughter and her husband
join the realm of the unknown.
She's on the move to more of the unknown.

We don't know what will happen next.
We're primed for action,
but we're never really ready.

Who knows what's next?
It's more of the unknown.

WE BOTH HURT

My sister has been in deep emotional pain.
Now she's in physical pain, too.
She has a bad case of the shingles,
and I am sure it's stress related.
How do I help her cope?
What can I do at this end?
I feel her pain, both physical and emotional.
As a caregiver at a distance, it eats me up too.
Does she know?
Does she care?
Is she so caught up in her own pain
that she can't see my pain?

I hurt for all of us.

NO ROOM

Dad's ready for help, to go to assisted living.
They've been waiting for months for an opening.
He needs help, he wants help, he is asking for help.
But there are no rooms available.

We wait and wait some more.
It's driving him crazy, the waiting.
What should have been weeks is now months.
Dad will take any opening now, anything.

He needs the help.
We need to find it for him.

What do we do when there is no room at the inn?

DAM HAS BROKEN

The dam has broken.
Her mind seems to be flooded
with the debris of her life.
There is no control now.
This is the flood.

She plunges into the darkest memory,
and brings up the detritus of her soul.
She rides the river, plunges in,
and is submerged in her anger, in her rage.
The waters boil up around her,
around us.

We're in a maelstrom.
How do we get out?
How does she?
The dam has broken.

God help us all.

DROWNING

Help me, I'm lost.
Help me, I'm falling.
Help me, I'm drowning.
Help me, I'm falling apart.

There is nothing left.
Help me find the pieces
before I go under.

WINTER IS COMING

It's almost Autumn.
Summer is ending and with it the sun showers.
We're getting more thunderstorms.
They frighten us,
more thunderstorms, more lightning.
Will any of us get struck?

The leaves are falling,
colors are dull and faded.
They're reminders winter is approaching,
the rains turn more icy.

Winter is coming,
preparing us for remembering,
giving us time to focus on days gone by.
Time to remember yesterdays,
time to fall into the numbness of the next season.

The last season.
The lost season.

NO LONGER HERE

Where did she go?
The woman she was is no longer here with us.
We'll get glimpses of her here and there.

My sister tries to explain to Dad about Mom's condition,
but he doesn't get it.
He thinks he can bring her back to him.
He thinks his unconditional love will reach out to her,
and bring her back.

She's too far gone.
She's lost.

He won't give up.
He wants her back.
He won't give up.

Should we?

GRANDMA AND GRANDPA

I visited my grandparents this summer,
and entered the pain of my grandmother's dementia.
She's gone away to another world.
I tried to bring her back,
"Grandma, remember our trip to Yellowstone?
Remember our trips to Raspberry Park?"
I loved to hear her tell me those stories.
I wish I could bring them back.
She tries.
But she doesn't get there.
I don't think she can go there anymore.

I watch my grandfather caring for her.
He wants to care for her, to do it himself.
That's what he expects of himself.
Not what we expect of him.
He can't do it anymore.
He is so stoic.
He would never let anyone see his frustration.
He loves her so much.
He's dealing with so much heartache.

I see the look on his face.
It's so sad.
He knows what is happening to Grandma.
He's so sad.
It's hard to watch him.
I am so sad.

It's frustrating to watch when she is agitated.
He doesn't know what to do.
He knows he needs help.
Sometimes I think he knows what he has to do next.
But he doesn't want to go there,
He knows he needs help.
We try.
It's so sad.

My grandma has turned into somebody else.
She is angry, so angry,
angry at everyone and everything.
She brings up names from the past
events from the past,
and seethes with anger.

Everyone tries to join her in her reality,
but she doesn't let us in.
I don't know what grandma is visually seeing.
It's like she's rented some movie
that none of us know about.

Grandpa is so frustrated.
Just the look on his face tells it all.
He wants his wife.
She's gone.

Grandpa calls his daughter, two, three times a night.
"Help me," he says. "I can't do this alone anymore."

Even though my aunt and uncle are there for them,
My grandparents need more.
They need more.

It's time for the move to assisted living.
Maybe even time for the nursing home.
They need more.

It's time.

RAINBOW

Rainbows are God's way of saying, "Hi there,
I am with you, even when you can't see me or feel me."

Today was a dark, cloudy, brooding day.
It was dark for my mother as she entered
into more loss of self.
Bleak and dark for my father and my sister,
and also for me.
I felt sad that I couldn't immediately help anyone,
not my sister, my father, and most of all my mother.
I felt caught up in the darkness.

And then I saw the rainbow,
a sign of God's promise, telling me,
"Hi there, I am with you."

Does Mom see the rainbow anymore?

TIDBITS

*"I need to take a bath,
I'm going to have a baby.
That's what I did before I had my first child."*

"Mom, you are ninety years old,
You are not having a baby!
Your body just feels a bit funny.
You are ninety years old!
You are not having a baby!"

She chuckles!

DARKNESS

In the beginning, the raging ocean covered everything
and was engulfed in total darkness.

My mother is a raging ocean that is engulfed in darkness.
It's not total darkness.
I hope there are glimpses of light,
glimpses of who she used to be.

God is with us as we move over the
raging waters of dementia.
Dear God, please let there be light!

LIGHTNING

My sister was almost struck by lightning,
She walked Dad to her car in a heavy rainstorm,
And on the way to the driver's side.
Crash! Bang! Lightning struck!
She threw herself into the car
as the smoking umbrella went flying!

It seems as if she's been struck over
and over by lightning.
Mom's dementia has accelerated,
and Dad gets weaker and more frail.
He calls and calls her for help,
and she is always there for them.

Stress has taken its toll,
and she suffers from a bout of shingles.
She really has been struck by lightning
and needs to jump into a safety net.
How about a cushion for her burdens?
something to help her
when she is in the driver's seat.

What can I do from here?
How can I be their lightning rod?

MORE THAN THEY CAN HANDLE

Mom has to stay another weekend in the hospital.
Her meds are not controlling her behaviors.
She still has paranoia and talks constantly.
It's taking longer to learn how to handle her.
Dad and my sister visit her every night.
They sit and listen to her chattering.
Sometimes she knows them and welcomes them.
Sometimes she tunes them out and goes on and on and on.
Nothing seems to be helping Mom.
She is still out of whack.

Dad wants to take Mom back home with him.
Can't he see that she is more than he can handle?
He made a promise that he would never leave her.
Can't he see that she has left him?
He had another lock put on the door to their apartment.
Can't he see Mom feels she is in a prison?
He wants to take care of her himself.
Can't he see she is more than he can handle?

My sister cannot go in the middle of the night to calm her.
She is totally stressed out.
Dad calls her two, three times a night when Mom is out of control.
Dad can't handle things anymore.
My sister can't handle things anymore.
Who can handle Mom now?

It is time.
Time for the nursing home.
Time for the Special Alzheimer's Care Unit.
Mom needs more.
They can provide it.
Will Dad let her go?
Who can handle Dad now?

DEEP WATER

We now are in deep water.
We don't know what the next wave will bring.
Will it crash over us?
Will we be able to ride it to shore?
We are in uncharted seas.

We are standing on the edge,
watching the waters of dementia toss her about.
It's as if our feet are glued to the sand,
and we can't get unstuck and go to her.

It's difficult to watch the waves knock her around.
Will she be able to come to shore again?
Will the next wave crash over her and sink her?

Or will the next wave crash over us
and sink us?

PRAYER

"Listen to my cry for help, for I am sunk in despair.
Set me free from my distress." Psalm 142, vs. 6.

Mom and Dad pray together every night.
Bedtime is prayer time,
prayers for thanksgiving,
for the gifts of love and life, family and friends,
special prayers for help and concerns.

Now I pray Mom's mind will find rest,
in all of the agony of her disbelief,
disbelieving who she is,
who Dad is,
who we are.

The Psalmist says, "Set me free from my distress."
I pray for my Mother's release from this captivity,
release from her disease that has captured her mind,
her thoughts, her memory, her self.
Release her.
Give her relief.

Give us all relief.

THERE IS ROOM AT THE INN

Mom and Dad are moving to assisted living.
Finally!
The wait is over.
We have lift-off!
Mom leaves the hospital and goes directly to the place.
She goes into a secured Alzheimer's unit,
and Dad goes into more independent living.
They will be together,
but not quite together.

Dad can visit her any time.
When she gets confused, angry, and frightened,
she will have caregivers to meet her special needs.
When he gets tired and needs some rest,
he can return to his own place.

This will be hardest on Dad,
to be away from her when she is 'out there.'
But then again, she has been 'out there' quite a bit lately.
Maybe it will be a relief to have Mom safe,
and have someone else directing and redirecting her.
It will be a relief to know he can have a full night's rest.

There will be people around them
to meet both their needs,
people around them to provide social times,
times to reminisce, and time to enjoy new things.
Hopefully Mom will respond to Dad's love,
and remember and recall their past history.
Hopefully Dad will begin to understand Mom's disease
by seeing others with the same symptoms.
Hopefully the professional caregivers will help
both of them adjust
so that their remaining time together will have some joy.

Hopefully we made the right decision
and we can help them adjust.
Aren't we the professional family caregivers?

SHE'S CHANGED

She's changed.
She's no longer the woman I married.
She's no longer the woman I had all those hopes and
dreams with.
She's changed.

Sometimes she doesn't even know me.
She doesn't remember our life together.
She's changed.

Sometimes it feels like she's died
and another person has entered her body.
It's not quite a death because I see her.
I talk to her.
But she's not there.
She's changed.

Sometimes she's home,
and I rejoice in having her back for awhile.
She leaves me more and more now.

She's changed.

I'VE CHANGED

I've changed too.
I can't seem to keep up with her anymore.
Not mentally or physically.
She moves too quickly for me to keep her safe.
I promised I would never leave her.

I've changed.
I have to leave her now.
Leave her for others to provide her care.

I've changed.
I can't do it alone anymore.
I need help.
I have help now.

I've changed.
I haven't left her.
We're both in the same place.
She's in a special unit
Where they can watch her every minute.
She's still with me every minute in my heart.
She's still a special part of my heart and soul.

It's hard to turn your heart over to someone else.
It's hard to put your head on the pillow
knowing your wife will never
put her head next to yours.
It's hard to say goodnight and walk away.
It's almost like saying goodbye.
I have to leave her now.

We've both changed.

RELIEF

Dad seems to find relief –
Relief from watching Mom every minute of every day.
He's torn.
On the one hand he is relieved,
on the other hand he feels guilt,
guilt over not being with her all the time,
guilt over having someone else provide her basic needs.
But he still provides the needs of the heart.
He still provides loving care through memories of a life
well lived together.
He shares in her care now.
When she has a bad day he can find some respite back in
his own place.
We hope he will make friends, enjoy the social times,
find some joy with others,
so that his life is not just broken memories of the past.
but a life reviewed and recognized as exceptional.
We think he's exceptional.

We feel relief too.

TIDBITS IN HUNGARIAN

I spoke to Mom after her first night in assisted living.
I spoke a few phrases in Hungarian.
Then I said goodnight, "jo' ejszakat."

She laughed and said to me,
*"What an elegant way you speak Hungarian,
how polished you sound,
I am so glad you remember your Hungarian."*

I am glad she remembers it too.
Mostly I am glad she remembered me!

ADMIRATION FROM A SON-IN-LAW

I admire you, Dad,
For your love and commitment,
Your devotion to Mom.
You're a role model for caring for a spouse who is ill.

I have a lot to live up to in following your lead.
You are truly a man who has lived
and followed his wedding vows.
You have always taken care of your family.
You have always taken care of your wife.

Now it's time to allow us to share in that care,
to share your commitment,
to share your pain,
to share our love and devotion.

MY RELIEF

When I visited their assisted living home,
I was relieved and pleased,
relieved that I can let them go to other caregivers,
relieved they will be there 24 hours a day,
relieved they will be safe,
relieved they will be with other people and not alone.
relieved they will have more opportunities.

I am pleased, so pleased,
pleased that the place is a lovely home,
pleased that the staff is so responsive to them,
pleased to see their own places,
pleased to see them in a routine already,
pleased to see the relief in my father's eyes,
pleased to see my mother be with my father
during the day,
pleased to see her in a special Alzheimer's unit at night,
pleased to see my father's relief.
pleased to see my sister's relief.

Pleased and relieved.

SEPARATE BUT NOT APART

It's hard to have them in separate rooms,
in separate parts of the building.
I know they don't like being apart,
yet it is a fact of their new existence.

Dad tucks Mom in at night, in the Alzheimer unit,
gets her into her nightgown,
reminds her to wash her face and brush her teeth,
just like he did to us when were young.

Now he takes care of her.
Sometimes she doesn't want his help,
doesn't acknowledge he's her husband,
doesn't respond to him.
In those times he gets so frustrated,
so hurt by her rejection of him.

Then he's glad he has a separate place for her,
someone to watch her and keep her safe for awhile,
someone to redirect her,
someone to walk with her
when she is restless in the middle of the night,
someone to listen to her
when she can't stop telling her stories,
someone else to cover for a time
so he can rest and recover
and in the morning pick her up
and start the day together in the hope,
hope that she is with herself,

and will be with him.

LOCKED AND UNLOCKED

I wish they were in an apartment together.
They have their separate places due to Mom's needs.
She can't spend the night with Dad.
It's too risky for her.
She may wander off.
So she sleeps in the Alzheimer's unit.
The doors are locked.
If she wanders,
she has lots of space in a secured spot.

But the days are with Dad.
He enters her area,
unlocks the code to the entrance,
and joins her.
He gathers her for the day to his place.

She unlocks the code to his heart,
if she is present in the now.
He rejoices in his wife being with him.
Together they pass the hours of the day,
sharing meals,
sharing memories,
sharing the time they have left,
unlocking each other's hearts and souls together.

DON'T LEAVE ME ALONE

*I don't like it when you leave me in this room.
I get scared being by myself.
It's cold sleeping alone.
What am I supposed to do for eight hours in this bed?
Don't leave me alone.*

I am scared.

I DON'T WANT TO BE ALONE EITHER

I don't like having you in that other place.
But I have to keep you safe.
I don't want to look out the window,
and see you roaming outside in your nightgown.
We need this place,
Both of us need to be here.
I can't do it alone anymore.
I am so tired.
And you need to be safe at night.
At least we can be together during the day.
And I can sleep during the night,
And be able to take care of you in the morning.
Don't think I have abandoned you.
Every morning I will be there for you.
And every night I will tuck you in.
After all, it's just eight hours
and we will be together again.

What's eight hours after a lifetime spent together?

ACCEPTING THE UNACCEPTABLE

After all Mom went through losing an eye,
suffering with cancer,
all the emotional pain she had dealing with in-laws,
you'd think that was enough suffering in a lifetime.
Shouldn't she be spared any more pain?

Then this disease strikes, this dementia.
It's like a cancer eating up her memory,
destroying her personality,
creating a stranger.

It's hard to accept the unacceptable.
We feel angry and even impotent.
We even feel mad at God for allowing this to happen.
This is a hard thing to accept.
We know that things happen to us,
and God gives God's strength, God's power,
God's love to sustain us.
Mom and Dad seem to be accepting this.
They don't understand why,
they just accept the unacceptable and go on.
Somehow Mom and Dad have found the faith and courage
to go on.

We must, too.

THE DOCTOR

How lucky did we get?
We have the best geriatrician in the state.
Mom and Dad are in good hands.
I sat in a session with him on the last visit.
I am so pleased.
He is gentle and kind and yet authoritative with them.
He knows how to work with elderly patients.
My parents like him as their physician.
That is half the battle.

At the last visit I attended,
he asked my Mom "Where is your husband?"
She replied, *"It better be this man next to me
as I came with him."*
He then asked her who he was,
And she laughed aloud and stated,
*"I hope you know who you are,
you are supposed to be my doctor."*

So far no great changes in their condition have occurred.
Mom's dementia has increased,
and Dad's cancer is stable.

So we go on,
one day at a time,
dealing with all the nuances of dementia,
dealing with all the nuances of aging.
dealing with all the nuances of caregiving.

We go on.

THE PAID CAREGIVERS

What would we do without the staff at Mom's place?
They take care of most of her needs.
From the time she gets up in the morning,
till she goes to bed at night,
they are there for her.
Dressing her, bathing, toileting her,
cleaning up after her messes,
they are there.

They bring her out of the locked area every other morning
to visit with Dad.
She spends some time in his apartment with him,
just being together.
Then it's down to the dining room for lunch.
They sit at a table for four and enjoy a meal together.
Sometimes she gets agitated,
And that makes it tough for Dad.
"He's staring at me", she says of their tablemate.

Dad tries to help her cope.
He knows when it's a bad day,
and he has to get her back to her area of the facility.
He tries to hold on to her for awhile after lunch,
so they can have some more time together.
But more often he calls
one of the girls to take her home to her place.
They come and gently bring her back to her other reality.
They are caring and respectful of both her and Dad.

The staff knows when Mom is especially agitated
or out of sorts.
Then they keep her at her place,
trying to find some activity for her to get involved.
They know her and her moods.
It's hard on Dad when she doesn't want to
come and visit him.

The staff at his end of the facility understand his dilemma.
They try to find ways to involve him in activities,
engage him in conversation, help him to build friendships.
They care about him too.

It's hard to turn over your parents to paid caregivers.
You turn over your trust to them,
and hope for the best.

Sometimes you get so angry about things not working.
Mostly it's about how fast they get to do
what needs to be done.
It's hard to share your parents with caregivers who have
other people to care for too.
You want the one-on-one care,
but realize that is not possible.
So you bend, you yield, you accept.
And just ask for people who will learn to like your parents,
with all their quirks,
maybe even learn to love them in time.

We are lucky with our parents' caregivers.
I think they like them.

I know I like the caregivers.

DON'T LIKE IT HERE

This is a big place, where we live now.
Mary is at the other end of the building.
I used to walk down there to meet her,
to bring her back to my place.
Our place is gone.
Now we have her place and my place,
that place and this place.

I am tired, so tired, to go and get her.
The girls bring her to my place.
Even when she's here in my place she's not here.
She's not in any place.
She's off in her own world.
I wish we were both in another world.
We're ready to go.

I don't like this place we're in,
the separation from each other,
the physical pain,
the loss.
I sure could talk about the losses!
I miss it all.
But most of all I miss Mary.
She's leaving me more and more each day.

How long before she completely goes?

COMMUNICATION

My sister dropped in to visit Mom on her unit,
and found her in deep conversation with another lady.
My sister thought, oh how nice for Mom to have
a friend to talk with.
As she approached them my sister found the other lady
babbling,
talking in nonsensical words.

Mom was talking with her in a conversational way,
and both ladies were having an enjoyable visit.
Somehow the two of them communicated,
sharing as two women face to face through time
have always done,
in the give and take of talking.

Mom recognized my sister as soon
as she approached them.
"Here's my daughter," she beamed.
She was overjoyed to see her daughter and introduce her
to her new friend.
My sister was overjoyed Mom recognized her.
That made her day, her week, her month.

Communication is wonderful when it occurs,
in whatever means.

COME ON IN, THE WATER'S FINE

The last visit this Spring was wonderful.
She knew my husband and me for the entire week.
*"Oh, here's my daughter and her husband
from Wyoming,"*
she informed her friends in her care unit.
She was delighted to see us and was a delight to be with.
Her sense of humor was turned on.
"Please come in and visit, the water's fine."
And it was.

Mom told me she loved this place,
this vacation resort they were visiting.
She missed doing more traveling, more sightseeing.
But she enjoyed the food, the people, the accommodations.
Dad told her their traveling days were now memories.
And they certainly have tons of wonderful memories
of trips taken, sights seen, people visited.
The water was fine.

We spent time on calm waters for this visit.
visiting her at her care facility,
spending time with Dad and Mom for coffee breaks,
having a special luncheon with them at their place,
enjoying dinners at my sister's home with them,
even having a fun visit at the doctor's office.

Her sense of humor was right on, there too.
After her doctor asked her about her children,
She looked over at me and said,
*"There's my daughter Patricia Mary Novak.
Pardon me, Patty, but you got old!"*

How we all chuckled at her comment!
She sparkled with good humor and smiles.

Yes, the water was fine.

CHIPPER MOM

On the last visit Mom was so chipper.
She told me, " *We're on vacation here, at this resort.*
We are enjoying our stay here.
Sometimes your Father is gone doing his thing,
but that's ok, I keep busy.
I like it here.
I get used to it here.
And your Father was here the day before.
I'll stick around here and see what happens.
You got to do something,
when you can do something."

She enjoys the vacation from her daily activities,
the daily activities of sorting through her memories,
trying to put together her thoughts,
working through her challenges,
both physical and mental.
Yes, she was on vacation when we visited this Spring.

It was a vacation for us too.

A GLORIOUS DAY

"Oh what a glorious day," she exclaimed.
She was happy, content with us visiting,
content with what was going on.
It was a glorious day for all of us.
How long will it last?

THE DANCE: A WALTZ IN ¾ TIME

How they did move in time to the dance music.
I loved watching them dance an old fashioned waltz.
They made it look so easy,
the one, two, three, one two three, turn two three.
They floated in each other's arms, dipping, swirling.
It was a beauteous thing to watch.

Their moves were in such synch.
How did they do it?
Years of practice, of trusting, of leading, of following,
of moving in tune to the music and to each other.

Their years together were a dance.
Dad always did the leading,
yet Mom allowed him to lead.
He controlled the movement,
and she gave in to the flow.
He supported her in the dips and swirls of the dance,
in the dips and swirls of their life together.

She made the dance look like a perfect piece.
They covered for each other.
When one faltered on a step, the other was there
to pick up the piece.
They were always there for each other,
picking up the pieces,
putting them together in new formations,
adding a new twist to the old pattern.

The old pattern doesn't exist anymore.
He tries to lead, but she doesn't remember the steps,
She can't follow anymore.
He gives a firm placement on her body
to guide her in the dance,
to help give her direction, to lead,
to hold her until she finds her footing.

She's lost her footing, can't find it anymore.
Sometimes she doesn't even remember who her partner is,
and resents the firm guidance he tries to give,
to lead her back into the dance.
I think they are done with the waltz.

She doesn't hear the sounds of that music

JITTERBUGS

We learned how to jitterbug watching Mom and Dad.
They would dance in the kitchen as the radio played a favorite tune.
Dad would come in the door and hear a bouncy beat,
take Mom in his arms and start to boogie.
"Wait a minute, let me take this apron off," she'd laugh.
He didn't care what she wore.
He heard the music of their early days
and took his lady for a spin around the room.
It didn't matter that it was in the middle of the kitchen.
All that mattered was Mom was in his arms,
and they were dancing to the beat.

They were so special to watch.
Wow, could they jive to the music!
My sister and I would laugh with them,
as they seemed to have so much fun dancing together.
Dad would let Mom go and grab onto one of us,
and then it was our turn to boogie.
We seemed to pick up the moves so easily,
probably, because we watched them so many times.
Dad would refine our moves, guide us,
lead us in the dance.
When it was our turn to dance, we boogied with style,
learned by following two of the best.

That's how we learned so many things from them both.
Dad would lead and Mom would follow his lead,
and my sister and I would watch and wait
until we were invited in.
Led by Dad, guided by Mom until we could be on our own,
was the way we learned the steps to life.
We practiced together as a family
until it was our turn to dance.

My sister and I never got the hang of letting
someone else lead us.
When we jitterbug together we laugh
as both of us try to lead.
I guess that's the story of our lives.
We only know how to lead.
We learned that from Dad in the dancing lessons.
Dad was the one in charge.
We weren't very good at following, like Mom.

He's not in charge anymore.
He's having to turn more and more over to us.
He can't jitterbug now.
His back and legs won't let him.
But oh the memories of that jiving music,
the memories of those moves, that rhythm,
the ebb and flow of the dance, the beat of the music.
He still has that.

I think it helps him
as he boogies with Mom on this river of dementia.

KARAOKE

Dad danced with Mom this week.
The facility had a karaoke presentation for an activity,
and they had a ball being part of the fun .
Dad sang "I left my heart in San Francisco".
and then asked his lady for a dance.
She refused at first,
so he sang the song again, just for her.
She got it!

They moved around the dance floor together.
Dad was a bit tentative,
watching out for his back and knees,
but they danced together!
Feeling the flow,
enjoying the movement,
loving the moment,
they danced.

They were a couple again for a time, dance partners,
husband and wife, partners for life,
rediscovered through the music of the dance.
They moved together with fluid movements,
remembered through years of practice.
Flowing smoothly,
they danced on the river of dementia.

What a joy it was for them both, in the dancing,
and in the sharing with us.
This was a moment for all of us to enjoy,
floating, flowing in sync,
while traveling on the river of dementia.

It was a smooth trip.

LESSONS TO LEARN

Mom and Dad are still teaching us,
with Dad's devotion and commitment to Mom,
with Mom's zingers,
bits and pieces of her humor, her pain.
We're learning a lot about some of Mom's past,
of some of her unresolved anger and pain,
her disappointments.

We're learning how to model caregiving
and be understanding of dementia,
to show our own children a way of living and loving,
of being there for each other no matter what.

Yes Mom and Dad are still teaching us.
And we are all learning together.

BENEDICTIONS

I say goodbye to Dad in his apartment,
"I don't know when I'll see you again."
He tells me,
*"That's ok,
We've had a good life together,
What will be, will be,
Go."*

I say goodbye to Mom in her room.
"Mom, I miss you so much."
She tells me,
*"I don't worry about saying goodbye anymore.
I don't dwell on it.
Don't let it hurt you.
Just go on and live your life.
Go on, go on,
And remember me."*

What will be, will be,

And I will never forget.

FOG HAS SETTLED IN

The fog has settled in.
It doesn't seem to lift off anymore.
We're all enveloped in grayness.
The fog has settled in.

Sometimes it's heavy and dense,
Sometimes light and filmy.
But it's still fog,
And the fog has settled in.

It's wet and raw now.
It doesn't lift off anymore.
No more sunshine.
The fog has settled in.

We don't know where she is anymore.
The fog has settled in.
We don't know where we are anymore.
The fog has settled in.

FILL YOUR POT

My dear sister,
Be gentle with yourself.
Allow others to nurture and care for you.
You are busy living a life serving others ,
serving your spouse and children's needs,
serving your school, staff, and students,
serving Mom and Dad's needs.
You need to stay in balance.
You need to serve yourself as well.

The other side of giving is receiving.
You need to reach out and ask for what you need.
This way you give others a chance
to reach out and help you,
paying back all the goodness you give to others.
Get your courage up and ask for support and help.
Ask for what you need.

Fill your pot, feed it girl!

THOUGHTS WHILE RETURNING ON THE PLANE

What's next?
What will happen next?
I look out at the horizon
But I cannot see beyond a certain point.
It gets foggy out there,
hazy, misty.
The plane wing tilts up, and then back down again.
Just like my parents' lives,
a tilt up, good things happen.
a tilt down, and they plunge into darkness.

We plunge and tilt with them.
As we tilt downwards, we see with more clarity
the reality below us.
And as we fly upwards, we see more sunshine
that will sustain us during those downward slides.

The edge of the horizon, all I can see is not the end,
but a beginning somewhere else.
My parents lives are tilting and plunging.
Yet I know there is a beginning somewhere else,
over the horizon,
over the next rainbow,
where God will be calling and saying,
"Hi there,
Welcome home."

BUMPY RIDE

It's cloudy now,
I cannot see the ground,
Just a sea of clouds as far as the eye can see.
It's a bumpy ride.
We're tossing and tilting.
We have to plunge through those clouds
To make a landing.
It will be a bumpy ride.

Mom and Dad, hang on.
It will be a bumpy ride.
Safe landing after the ride.

Safe landing to your final home.

MY SEPARATION

Upon landing, I have really left my parents.
I have said goodbye.
While in the air I was connected to them, in limbo,
somehow closer to them up there.
Now I am on the ground
and feeling the reality of the separation.
I don't like being so far away.
But I am so close to them in my heart.
My heart is never locked to their love.

IN THE MIDST OF THE WHIRLWIND

Today a tornado came through town in the middle of the afternoon.
While sitting at a local restaurant
we heard the sirens go off,
and were directed to a safe area in the hotel/restaurant.
We watched the torrential rains, wind, and then the hail.
We knew what would come next.
So we gathered with other patrons in an inside room,
waiting.

It's exhausting, this waiting,
wondering when and if it will hit.
The word was it was heading to our home neighborhood.
Already reports arrived about trucks turned over,
roofs blown off, and signs and poles blown down.
We were hunkered down in a safe area,
wondering about our home,
waiting for the all clear call
so we could go home and check,
waiting, wondering, worrying.

It's like that with my Mom and Dad.
We are waiting, wondering, worrying
when the cancer will take Dad,
when the dementia will take Mom.
It's exhausting, this waiting,
wondering not if, but when it will hit.

Sometimes I feel as if I am hunkered down too,
waiting, wondering, worrying,
being in a place not of my choosing,
a place where I have to sit and wait
until I hear something definite.

That's what care giving at a distance feels like,
being in a place not of your choosing,
waiting for a word to come and be there,

wondering if you can do anything in a short visit,
worrying that you are not doing enough,
knowing that you cannot be there due to circumstances
you cannot control,
worrying that you cannot do enough,
knowing that their 'roof' can be blown off any second,
that their lives will be turned upside down,
and the poles and the direction markers of their
relationship and yours are shattered.

There is no safe area in which to hunker down.
We are caught out in the middle of the tornado,
blown apart, with stinging rain
and hailstones pummeling us.
Like being in the middle of the storm,

and waiting for the tornado to come and shatter us.
We are now in the midst of the whirlwind.

A SHIFT

I lost it today.
It hit me hard about losing my parents.
They are still alive,
but I am losing them.

I got back from my Mother's Day visit with them,
and tried to get back in the groove,
with my job, my life here.
Then the tornado hit,
and my emotions were as cyclonic as the wind.
Two days of no electricity, no water, no heat,
no regular life.
Winds, rains, hails and then snow,
we got hit by it all,
and so did I,
hit by it all.

The tornado symbolized my turbulent life.
It's as if I have been thrown to the winds,
buffeted about with everything that could fall from the sky,
and then left with picking up the pieces.
The pieces don't seem to be in the same places anymore.
There has been a shift.
Nothing seems to fit.
Things are not the way they were.
There has been a big shift,
and I can feel the change.

I feel lost.
It is beyond my control.
I hope it is not beyond my endurance.
I hope I can go on.
With God's grace and God's presence in my life,
I will go on.

I will try.

CHECKING UP AFTER THE TORNADO

Traveling from a distance to visit is like checking up after a tornado.
You don't know what you will see, what you will encounter.
Their physical selves have changed, and their bodies become more frail.
They become more bent over from all the physical ailments,
from all the emotional burdens they carry,
like trees in a tornado, not yet uprooted, but damaged,
wondering if they will be able to still stand,
not quite upright.
How many more blows will the old trees be able to withstand and survive?

My parents have survived so many difficulties and problems.
They have handled obstacles as minor annoyances, inconveniences.
It's not just discomfort anymore,
it's distress.
It's with a sense of sadness that they view their circumstances.
They do not have an 'adjuster' to determine what can be fixed,
what can be replaced.
They hold on and hope they can continue to function,
while battered and bruised by the tornado
that entered their lives.

I came to visit after the last tornado blew through,
checking, assessing, evaluating, redirecting,
trying to figure where we are now,
what direction we are heading,
where we are going to be next.
They don't see how weakened they are after the storms.
They don't see the need for any more props
to hold them up,

to support and strengthen them,
to keep them functioning at their present abilities.

But we do.
My sister and I asked for more assistance from their
facility,
to prop them up in a way that
doesn't undermine their pride.
We figured a way to negotiate with them
and give them choices,
choices to help them survive in their weakened conditions.
We hope we are at a plateau and can take a breather.
We know they are hoping for that too,
a breather,
before the next tornado hits.

SHUFFLING OFF

She walks, shuffling her feet,
holding on to the ground.
Her reality is to touch base while walking,
to hold on to something stable, something sure.
She's afraid to pick up her feet and lose that security.
I hold on to her to give her a secure base.
Roles are now reversed.
She doesn't hold my hand.
I hold hers and lead her.

I remember all the times I held her hand to be safe.
I trusted her to take care of me.
I would run to keep up with her,
she walked so much faster than me at times.

Now she moves shuffling, moving slowly.
She doesn't know where she is going.
Sometimes she doesn't know who is leading her,
guiding her.
When she knows us, knows Dad,
she trusts by holding a hand,
a warm hand that wraps around her
and wraps around our hearts.

AFTER FALLING OFF THE BUS

Coming back to their facility Mom fell
while getting off the bus.
She lost her balance and fell backward.
Crash! Bang!
She hit her head hard on the concrete.
She was stunned physically and mentally.
Staff took action and got her to the hospital ER.
Dad was a nervous wreck,
sitting, waiting, watching, worrying.
It took awhile to receive care,
but it was nothing serious.
So back to the facility with some bed rest and Tylenol.

NOTHING SERIOUS?
Who are they kidding?
This is serious stuff here.
She fell completely backwards and jarred her head.
She doesn't need any more damage to her brain!

We are all stunned,
having been caught off balance,
just like Mom.
Who knows what will happen next.

Each day is an adventure for both Mom and Dad.
Each day is a trip to an unknown destination.
We are always waiting, watching, worrying,
to hear about the next day's journey,
hoping it was a pleasant one,
and not another
Crash! Bang!

SHE'S NOT HERE, DAD'S LAMENT

Oh my God, she's not here.
Where did she go?
I had her in my room, watching TV.
I guess I dozed off.
I thought the girls had come for her,
to get her dressed for our party.
I went to her locked unit.
She wasn't in there.
I went upstairs to the party.
She wasn't there either.

Now I got worried.
I figured she's been gone for a while now.
I told the girls, my Mary is gone.
I can't find her anywhere in the building.
So they searched for her,
upstairs and down, inside and out.
They can't find her.
Now I am getting scared.
She's not here, she's really gone.

I know she's been leaving me bit by bit.
This is different.
She is really gone.
Where are you, Mary?
Where did you go?
What did I do?
I fell asleep, that's what I did,
and she quietly opened the door and left.
Mary don't leave me yet,
not like this,
not like this.

They found her!
Thank goodness, they found her!
They found her walking along the highway,
far away from here.

How did she get that far away?
She shuffles when she walks in here.
They tell me she was moving fast,
striding through the grass.
Thank goodness they found her!

Where was she going?
Why was she running away?
Why was she running from here?
Why was she running from me?
Why? Why? Why?
I have so many questions,
but she can't tell me the answers.
I love you, Mary.
I want you with me.
I don't want to lose you,
not like this,

not like this.

SHE'S EDGY AND HE STILL LOVES HER

Mom was confused again and edgy - angry.
I could not engage her in any bit of conversation.
She was mad and negative.
After trying and trying I visited with Dad.

Dad just keeps on keeping on.
He is in denial about how far she's gone.
I don't think he can acknowledge how far
and how lost she is.
I think he needs to hold on to her every second,
or she will really disappear from him and from us all.
The routine of their days is important to him.
He is so full of joy when he picks her up from her locked
unit, and has her for the day.

She looked like a bag lady today
when he brought her to his apartment.
Her hair wasn't combed, and she looked disheveled,
wearing pants that didn't fit and a sweater too baggy
to be her clothing.
I fix her hair and adjust her clothing
to make her presentable.
She mumbles and mumbles, is barely coherent.
She doesn't want to talk about anything and tells me so.

Dad sits and smiles at her and tries to get a response.
It's beautiful to see the love Dad feels for her.
She is his life, always has been.
He wants to be with her every minute
of the life together they have left.
He knows she is vulnerable and he wants to protect her.
He feels the need to make some semblance
of their marriage,
their life together, by being there for her.

This summer they will have been married for 68 years.
Dad is so proud of that.

He accepts everything from Mom,
He accepts her as she is.
His love forgives and accepts and takes each day as a gift.
To him, she is beautiful, just as she is.
When she smiles, he beams with joy.

How can I separate them more?
It will crush him.
Yet Mom needs to be in a safe, secured place.
Being in that place, makes Dad
see what she will become like.
So he wants to keep her with him.
He thinks by keeping her with him all the time,
he can hold on to her,
keep her surrounded by his love and his memories.
Maybe she will respond to a memory
of their lives shared together.
He accepts the crumbs she offers.
Sometimes it is a delicious offering
of remembered moments shared in joy.
So he tries.
He lives for those moments.
He will take them when they come.

How I wish I could bring my Mom back to my Dad.
I wish I could share more than having a meal together,
a walk in the garden, a walk inside the facility.
I wish for more time for her to recall their special
moments.

But I have to accept what is, and go on back to my life.
I say goodbye to them and help walk Mom back to her unit.
I say, "I love you, Mom."
She looked at me and said, *"I love you too, Patty."*
So for that I am thankful.
I had my Mommy for a bit more.

She will always have me for her daughter,
and she will always have my Dad for her loving husband.
We will hold the loving memories of her in our hearts.

MOTHER'S DAY

It was wonderful to be with Mom for Mother's Day.
I can't be there on a day to day,
or even a weekend to weekend basis,
so I took a week's time to be there now.

I saw firsthand the problems with which my sister deals,
like Dad's worries and concerns about his bills,
(that's undaunting for anyone at any age,
let alone a 92 year old),
like Mom's difficulty in leaving her known area,
and just traveling to my sister's house,
her confusion, her car sickness, her anger.

I was there and sometimes so was Mom.
So I took what she gave and she accepted my gifts.

My sister and I gifted her with a Hungarian dinner,
accompanied by Hungarian Gypsy violin music.
We served up stuffed cabbage, cucumber salad,
and rye bread,
kifli cookies and palacsinta crepes for dessert,
all on Mom's good china, her crystal and silver.
"This looks familiar," she said.
It was a celebration of all the Hungarian dinners
she served us,
every Sunday after church.
The only thing missing was the chicken soup!

It was a good day for her and for us.
It was a time she knew us.
We looked familiar too.
Our daughters were also with us, her two granddaughters.
They look familiar to her too.
It was a good day.

I had a Mother for Mother's Day.

HE JUST KEEPS ON KEEPING ON

Dad just keeps on keeping on.
He is in denial about how far Mom has gone.
I don't think he can acknowledge how far she has gone,
how lost she is.

He feels he has to hold on to her every second,
or she will really disappear,
and leave us all mentally.

He gets so overwhelmed with all the paperwork, the bills.
My sister helps here.
Dad is trying so hard to keep it all together.

The routine is critical to him,
routine with Mom,
routine with bills and notices of insurances.
He needs to handle the bills, finger the papers,
to get a grip on what it's all about.

How can we help him get a grip about
what Mom is all about?

DOWN THE HIGHWAY FOR A WALK

She's lost.
This time for over two hours.
She left the facility and went for a walk,
down toward the action,
down the avenue to the highway.
She couldn't find a sidewalk, so she stuck to the grass.
On and on she walks.

"Is this the way home?" she thought.
*"Maybe if I keep going, I'll find the way,
find my way.
Uh oh, I think I'm way off course.
This is definitely not the way.
Where is my way?
Where is MY WAY?"*

On and on she walks,
on and on and on and on.

DEPENDS

I am numb.
It's hard to say goodbye after a visit,
not knowing when or if I will seen them again.

Dad is so frail and tires more.
Using the walker he has to slow down, stop,
take a breath every now and then.
He gets winded, and his arms hurt,
with the weight of using the walker.
He doesn't want to be dependent on it,
and walks short distances without it.
He parks it in his apartment,
and hold on to chairs, the bed, the dresser, the walls.
He tries so hard to maintain his independence, his dignity.

Depends

He started to wear incontinence pads.
Thank goodness for that product,
but he's developed a rash on his genitals,
probably not changing the Depends often enough.
He says they are not wet through,
so he puts them back on after a bathroom trip.

Depends

My sister and I went to the pharmacy
and asked what to do.
They said he needs to change the pads more often.
We also bought some antibiotic cream and powder,
and told him how to use them.
Hope it helps him.

Depends

We can't believe we, his daughters,
are telling him how to deal with jock rash
from wearing diapers.
We laugh over it with him.
But inside we are crying.

DAD'S BIG THREE

We had to move away from all we knew,
our home, our friends, our church, clubs.
Everything that was familiar to us after a lifetime of living
in one place.
That was the hardest thing for me.
This was the place of birth, my schooling, my work.
It was the place for the two of us as newlyweds, as parents.
It was a time and place where we built a life.
It was our life.

Then we just got old and frail,
couldn't do it alone anymore.
Our daughters said it was time to move,
to live near one of them.
Do we go to the mountains with all its snow?
with the high altitude and cold?
Or do we go down South where it gets so hot,
and deal with the humidity and the bugs?

I remember visiting out West
and having trouble breathing.
That high altitude is rough on your heart and lungs,
especially when you are old and not used to it.
I was sick and tired of all the snow we had in Jersey.
Couldn't live in a place that had more snow to deal with.
I am too old to shovel, and it's hard to find help these days.

So we moved down South.
It's not our home, but it's where we live now.
At least we were together for a while.
Now we live in the same building,
just at opposite places.

I miss Mary, sharing our lives together.
At least I get to be with her on her good days.

THE SECOND THING I MISS

The second thing I miss is driving.
We loved to go out together for a ride,
just to get out of the house, see some scenery,
a visit to old familiar places, to new sights.
I loved driving, just the feel of the wheel in my hands.
After all I did work for Ford Motor Company.
Driving was one of my joys.

At first I gave up driving at night.
I had trouble with all the bright lights, the glare.
It was time to give up the night.
Moving to a new place became a challenge to me.
I didn't have all the familiar signs and
places to connect me.
I seemed to get lost so easily.

You had to drive to get anywhere, for anything.
I know I complained about how far I had to drive to find
stuff.
I think it was an excuse for how hard it was
to find where I was going.
I got lost a lot of times.
Of course I blamed it on poor directions,
no signs to help me out.

And then I had the problem with my 'going problem.'
I always had to find a place to 'go.'
I put a coffee can and then a urinal device in the car,
just to be safe in a pinch.
It got harder and harder to go for a ride,
without using my emergency equipment.

And then I knew I wasn't as quick to deal with things.
I had a few close calls.
Didn't want to tell my girls, but I think they knew.
I couldn't hide it when they were with me in the car.
It got difficult to drive with Mary in the car.

I had to watch out for her,
watch out she didn't open the door and try to leave,
watch out she didn't open the window and throw stuff out,
like the hearing aid she thought was a bug in her ear.
If I stopped for a break,
I was afraid she would leave the car.
Her dementia scared me.
It was time to stop driving.
Time to stop driving, time to sell my car.

It was time.
Yes, it was a 'time' for me."

NUMBER THREE TO DEAL WITH

I have lost my walk.
Can't seem to make these old legs go like they used to.
I spent a lifetime on them.
I was not a desk jockey.
I was a mover and shaker.
I used these old legs walking up and down stairs,
I was never still, always on the move.

These legs got me my lady.
Met her at a dance and spent the
rest of our lives dancing together.
We danced together for almost 68 years.
These legs could waltz, fox trot, lindy, and jitterbug.
These old legs could tell you stories.

Now they don't work so good.
I tried a cane for a while,
but I can't use it anymore.
Hurts my shoulders to lean on it.
I am not safe without some help.
Can't help myself like I used to.

So it's time to use a walker.
This is a souped up model,
with brakes and a seat.
But it's still a walker,
and I have to use it to go anyplace.
I got old.

I don't like to be dependent.
But I still want to be independent.
So the walker it is.
I just have to look at it as getting my walk back.
I think I can handle that.

GOING DOWNHILL

Mom isn't the only one going downhill.
Dad is diminished too,
diminished in stature from his spinal stenosis,
diminished in stamina from his aging and the cancer,
diminished in mental reasoning from being stressed and
overwhelmed.

He's tired, so tired.
But he won't give in.
He has to care for Mom.
He can't let her get away.
He holds on to her physically and emotionally.
He tries to keep her grounded in his love.
He can't let her get away.

They don't spend their nights together.
She sleeps in a locked unit for safety's sake.
He keeps her with him most of the day,
and holds on to her.
He can't let her get away.

He savors the moments when she is lucid,
and remembers him and their times together,
in a shared life of loving and living.
He winks at her and she winks back,
a connection,
a spark.
He can't let her get away.

Oh, how his love reaches out to her.
How he tries to get a response, a spark from her.
How overjoyed he is by her response.
It keeps him going,
when she has bad days, when she is angry,
when she stubbornly refuses his care,
refuses him.
He can't let her get away.

It is a beautiful sight to see them walking together,
hand in hand.
What glorious love,
what glorious commitment.
He holds on to her and won't let her get away.

SHE WON'T LET ME IN

Sometimes Mom looks at me and doesn't see me.
I am a stranger to her.
She is not taking me in.
I try to reminisce about her memory times.
She won't let me in.
She is not taking me in.
I try to talk about special holidays,
the cooking, the baking.
She won't let me in.
She's not taking me in.

"Leave me be," she says.
Anger rides on her face,
in the crossed arms,
in the tilt of her chin.
She won't let me in.
She's not taking me in.

She's pushing me out,
pushing me away.
She won't let me in.

"I'm old," she says,
*"Old people don't want to talk about that,
I don't want to remember."*

She gets angry.
She's not taking her in either.

*"Why do you ask me to remember?
I don't want you to bug me.
Leave me be.
Leave me alone.
I'm not that person anymore.
I don't know who I am anymore.
You talk about this,
you talk about that,*

but I don't remember.
I can't remember!
Leave me along.
LEAVE ME ALONE!

I don't like it here.
I want to go home.
I'm tired.
I want to go home.
I'm too old.
I want to go home.
Please let me go home.

HOW CAN IT BE LIKE THIS

"How can it be like this?" she asked me.
"It's not here, it's not there."

She lost her memory and can't find it today.
She is confused and knows she is confused.
It is time for us to leave her,
and I am feeling so guilty, so sad.

"How can it be like this?"

HURRICANES

Hurricane Hanna is approaching Charleston
and I have to fly in.
The other storms are lined up waiting their turn
to create havoc on the shore.
Gale force winds are predicted.
You know what that means,
flying debris, storm damage, flooding.
This storm could intensify and create more chaos,
decreased visibility, increased turbulence.

How much more turbulence can we take.
This storm's track is uncertain.
Difficult to follow it on the radar.
Where will we go for shelter?
Who will rescue us?

How can I fly into this place?
What if I can't get there?
How will I deal with my turbulence?

Who will rescue me?

DAD IS FIGHTING THE CURRENT

I feel like I'm being carried by a current I cannot fight.
Sometimes I feel like I want to let it take me along,
and let it overtake me.
Maybe that way I will be set free.

But not yet, not yet.
There are too many things to get in order first.
How will I be able to do it all?
Will there be enough time before I succumb
to my own current?

FALLING BACKWARD

She has a hard time placing her body
where she wants it to go.
Just the other day she turned and fell over backwards.
He has such a hard time getting her back up.
He can't do it alone anymore.
So he calls for help.

She is on a downward fall into dementia.
She moves too fast and down she goes.
She turns and there she goes again.
When she walks she holds her feet to the ground,
and leans over watching where they go.
She's more stooped.
It's as if she needs to see the ground, watch it,
to know she is still connected to it.

He is still connected to her.
His love is a ribbon that encircles them,
leads them, covers them.
It's just that she trips over that ribbon,
doesn't see it,
misses it.

Oh he misses it too.
Misses the affirmation of their life together,
their years of loving and living,
her recognition of the ties that bind them.
He holds on tightly.
He won't let go.
As long as he is able,
he will hold her up.

Who will hold him up?

FALLING

She's now falling all the time.
They were sitting on the porch rockers
when she decided to go inside.
She fell on top of Dad and pushed him to the ground.
He couldn't get her to move off of him.
He tried to tell her to move her arms and legs.
She didn't know what to do.
There she was, on top of him.
Holding him to the ground,
crushing him into the hard concrete,
until someone found them and helped them.

It seems that she is crushing him, holding him down.
He's trying so hard to take care of her, to protect her,
to ease her way through her dementia.
So he cushions her,
with his body, his mind, his heart.

He gets hurt both physically and emotionally.
We try to ease his physical pain.
It's much harder to ease his emotional pain.

Who will cushion and protect him?

SISTER IS FALLING

This Fall my sister's life seemed to be falling,
falling downward,
falling apart,
falling into a whirlpool of unrest and unease,
of dismay and fear.

Her job has become more stressful.
She doesn't seem able to cope much anymore.
She seems to fall apart at the drop of a hat.
Then her husband had back surgery,
with a slow recovery.
Her daughter's Lupus has flared up,
with escalating pain.
Her son has suffered three seizures in six weeks,
with unknown etiology.
He falls for some unknown reason.
They are adult children, independent,
but still they are her children,
and she worries about their falling.
She's falling apart.
They all seem to be falling apart.

I go back in the Fall for a visit.
I help in the best way I can,
even though it's a short time.
I take Mom and Dad to their doctor's appointment,
trying to piece together their conditions,
trying to figure out what might happen next,
trying to predict when another fall could occur,
another fall into the downhill slide of dementia.

I celebrate Dad's 92nd birthday,
cook and bake in his honor.
cook and bake for my sister, too,
food for the table,
food to try to feed her tired spirit,
food to try to help heal her pain.

I can't do much to feed her tired spirit.
I listen and give sisterly advice.
I am there for her,
even when I am not there physically.
All I can really give her is my unconditional love,
to help cushion the falls.

FULL BODY ARMOUR

It seems like I have to be strong for everyone,
So I've armored myself well.
I have covered myself head to toe
with insulating, self-adjusting tons of steel.

The trouble is, I can barely keep my head above
the waters of the River of Dementia.
I have armored myself well,
so well, that I find myself sinking.

I can barely keep my own head above the water line,
let alone helping the rest stay afloat.

I don't like being strong for everyone.
It's a heavy load to carry.

WITHDRAWAL

Mom is withdrawing from everything outside herself.
She's going inside and sorting out,
evaluating her life.
As she processes her life,
she has shown anger.
There has been much in her life that was not in her control.
So now she is angry at the losses.
She retreats inside to process.
There is only room for her there.

It's as if she has a foot in two worlds,
her memory time,
and her present time.
She talks about people long gone and thinks we are them.
She is losing her grounding to us, to this time and place.
She has much unfinished business to accomplish,
and needs to validate these events and feelings.

When she finishes,
will she be finished with us?

MOM'S HANDS

The last time I visited I asked Mom to hold my hands
and make my achy pain go away.
She took my hands in hers and stroked them,
caressing away my pain.
It brought back memories of how her hands
soothed and calmed me,
during times of bruises, falls and even emotional pain.
I remember her hands reaching down to me,
holding on to me,
whenever we went walking,
holding on to me as we crossed streets,
guiding me along the way.

Her hands held my sister and me,
and enjoyed holding grandchildren
and even great-children.
Those hands clapped for us during performances,
awards and programs.
Those hands clapped in time to Broadway shows,
musical performances, plays.
Those hands held on to Dad's as they danced
through their lives together.

My Mother's hands were also tools.
She used them to form dough, cut out cookies,
for slicing, dicing, mixing, creating magic.
She was never afraid to tackle any culinary task.
It was as if she needed to touch the ingredients,
to gather them together,
to mix and meld a masterpiece of delight.
She had magic in her hands.
I treasure her handwritten recipes with
extra advice added to them.

Those hands were always fixing my hair,
rolling my hair in rags for baloney curls,

using Bobbi pins and hair rollers.
Her hands tried so hard to make my straight hair curly,
after my braids were cut.
Her hands showed me how to use my first lipstick.
I watched her hands 'fix her face',
and then use Pond's cold cream to take it off.
Her hands spritzed on her favorite perfume, and even
sprayed a bit on me.
I always think of her whenever I smell Arpege.

Her hands were working hands, too.
Her hands used a scrub brush and pail to do the floors.
She said that was the best way to do the cleaning,
on your hands and knees.
She made sure my sister and I learned
her methods of cleaning!
Her hands typed and noted numbers in her 'real' job,
working at the bank.
Her hands held the phone and took orders from my
father's customers
at the job she had when she came home from the bank.

Wherever I lived away from home,
I received letters from her hand.
At camp, at college, and in my own home after marriage,
She continued to write, describing the sights and sounds,
all the new places she and Dad visited.
It was her hand that held the maps
and Trip Tiks from AAA, to help Dad
navigate on our vacation trips.
She loved to write letters and describe all that she saw on
her many travels with Dad.
She encouraged us to write postcards to family and friends,
even when we had to ask her to spell every word.
Now I treasure every note, every card.
There will be no more written words from her.
I suppose these writings are a postcard to her
and from her.

Her loving, magical hands cared for all of us.
Now she is in the hands of the caregivers
at the Assisted Living,

and in the care of Dad's hands.
It is still a thrill to see Mom and Dad walking together,
Holding hands, holding on to the time they have left.

We know she is in God's hands,
And his hands will lovingly care for her,
Until he reaches for her hands to take her home.

GREATER OR LESSER, THEM OR THOSE PEOPLE: IT DEPENDS ON YOUR VIEW

I have never given much thought to
the possibility of me getting dementia.
That is until now.
Now that my Mother has Alzheimer's disease
it is a real possibility.
The odds that I will have some kind of memory loss is real,
very real now.
I turn 65 in a few days.
The statistics say 10% of those over 65 will have
some form of dementia.
That increases to over 47% of 85 year olds.
And with a parent with the disease the odds are greater.

Greater?
I wouldn't call it any form of great!
If anything, it's lesser.
It diminishes a person,
makes them less of who they were.

It seems as if we talk about them in past tenses,
talking about who they were and
not who they are anymore.
Who they are, has changed.
Who they were, is all we can hold on to.
And we hold on so tightly,
afraid to even lose that much of them.

That's why my Father is trying so hard to hold on to Mom.
That's why he hurries her out of her Alzheimer's unit,
and brings her to his place.
He tries to hold on to her, by keeping her tuned in to him.
He is so afraid she will turn into one of 'those people,'
who live on the Alzheimer's unit.

He doesn't get it.

She already is 'one of those people.'
It gets confusing,
'them,' 'those people.'
Depends on your point of view.
Depends on what part of the river you're viewing,
the river of dementia.

HE NEEDS TO DRINK, DRINK, DRINK

Dad had a trip to the ER hospital today.
He was too tired to go to the dining room for breakfast,
and told staff he wasn't hungry for lunch.
The staff figured out something was amiss,
and checked again.
He had an accident and was embarrassed.
They realized something was wrong
and sent him to the hospital.

Thank goodness my sister Janice was able
to go to the hospital,
And wait it out with Dad while all the tests were run.
Results came back with a report of bladder infection
and pneumonia.
My sister asked the doctor to keep Dad in overnight,
and check out if he had a stroke.

No stroke!
Thank goodness for that.
Dad needs to drink more liquids.
This is very hard for him
as he has to be near a bathroom a lot.
That's why he hasn't been going on van rides at the facility.
This is a huge embarrassment for him,
to be alert for a bathroom wherever he goes.

Janice had to deal with another huge embarrassment.
The doctor asked Dad to pee in a urinal,
and he couldn't do it himself.
Jan had to bite the bullet and help him..
This was a big, big embarrassment for them both.
They survived with a bit of humor.

That's how we all survive,
with a bit of humor.
Now the roles are reversed,
we are the ones in charge,

and they have to defer to us.

I hope we can all get through this.
We will have to find the solutions,
Find the humor and laugh.
What's the alternative?
We are doing enough crying!

ICE AGE

She's frozen in time,
locked in an iceberg.
She doesn't seem to feel much emotion.
She's on the river locked in ice,
tumbling down the river,
crashing into the banks,
feeling no pain,
having no notice of who she hits, who she hurts,
having no real idea of what's happening.
We can't seem to chip off the ice
to get to the real warm person she was.
She's frozen in time.

Her thoughts are frozen too.
Bitter cold emanations pour off her,
chilling us all to the bone.
She freezes us out.
Occasionally the sun comes out
and melts off some of that ice.
Then she feels, she sees, she knows.
It doesn't last long,
that sunshine, that warmth.
It doesn't take long for her to be iced up again.
Back to being frozen in time.
Cold – cold - so cold.

She's frozen in time.

BOULDERS AND SNAGS

Are we the boulders in her path on the river of dementia?
Do we stand in the way as she travels this route?
Are we the ones who stop her, stall her, to engage her?
Do we slow her down on the slide into dementia?
The boulders are bigger, now.
They hurt when she plows into them.
These memories are painful, these slips hurt.
She goes under and stays longer submerged in her deep dementia.

Or are we the snags that jut into the river
and entrap the river runner?
Do they say, "Stay, stop for a while, take a breather,
visit with us."
Are they a lifeline we throw out to her,
for her to grab onto?
Sometimes she does, most times she ignores us.
Or if she grabs on, it's to pull us along with her.

We're in danger of drowning too.
The water falls over deeper boulders, some hidden to us.
Sometimes she's trapped in an eddy,
With a memory she can't quite let go of.
Then she lets go and gets pulled into the white water.

There she goes, running the river.

ODE TO MY SUPPORT GROUP

My thanks to you my support group family.
You support me, hold me up, keep me grounded,
laugh with me, cry with me.
I couldn't survive without you.
You are awesome.
You are my lifeline.

Yes, I am the facilitator.
Yes I am in charge.
I see to your questions and concerns.
I bring you knowledge,
(after all I did chair the
State's Alzheimer's Association board).
I was their educator.
I know my stuff.
I've been leading a support group for over twenty years
now.

It's different when you have a
family member with dementia.
I know all about Alzheimer's in my head.
But I also know it in my heart.
Oh, boy, do I know it in my gut,
dealing with my parents' needs,
my sister's concerns.
I'm traveling with you on that River of Dementia.

We share stories of our rides.
Sometimes we are crashing onto the shores,
feeling so much pain as we take
the brunt of our caregiving.
Other times we feel we are drowning,
and can barely keep our heads above the water.
We help each other stay afloat.
and throw out lifelines,
to connect us to our loved ones,
and to each other.

You tell me how you survive,
and I tell you how I am surviving.
We do it together,
laughing, crying,
sharing anger, frustrations,
and yes even some of our joys.
Stories of how we coped,
how we are trying to cope now.

I've always felt that none of us is as smart as all of us.
And that's certainly true with our group.
Some of you have been with me for ages.
Others come and go as your needs come and go.
We welcome new members to our group,
and throw out the lifeline to each other.
Thank you for being my lifeline,
as we travel the River of Dementia.

I DON'T LIKE THE WATER

I never liked being on water, in water.
And here I am -
up to my neck in water.
It's cold and it's moving fast,
pulling me fast – faster.
I don't like being in the water.
My brother fell in the water and drowned.
I couldn't get him out.
And now I don't know how to get out.
I see people, hear their voices,
calling, yelling,
trying to grab me,
trying to reach me.

I don't think they can reach me anymore.
Sometimes I know who they are,
Sometimes I know who I am.
I think that's my husband.
Could that be my daughter?
I am moving faster now.
I can't grab on to them.
I'm trying - I'm trying.

The water is too fast, too cold.
It's got me now.
Will it pull me under?
I don't want to drown.
I don't like the water.
Help me get out of the water.

Is this the only way?

ROLLING ON THE RIVER

Be prepared for what will come.
Just how do we do that?
How do we prepare for her decline, her demise?
We're talking her death here.
How do we prepare?

The facility called and told us about her weight loss.
It's a roller coaster ride with her weight.
When we moved Dad and Mom from New Jersey,
she had lost about 25 pounds.
My sister and I thought that was the beginning of the end.
Then she entered the assisted living place,
ate three squares a day plus dessert and snacks.
Lo and behold she gained the 25 pounds back
plus a few more.
That was not the beginning of the end.

The extra weight helped her keep going.
She is still the energizer bunny and goes and goes,
not quite as fast or as often as when she first arrived.
Now she walks slower, sits more often.
So why is she losing weight?
Could be she is entering the stage of dementia,
where her body doesn't take on the pounds,
doesn't process all that food?
Her body is starting to say,
"Hey wait a minute – we're tired too,
tired of all that remembering, all that thinking,
all that confusion about who and what and where.
all that confusion of what to do,
of who I am today,
of who you are today."

Yes, it may be that time.
And then the roller coaster ride may take another rise,
another twist, another turn,
before it drops us all to the bottom
of the river we're rolling on.

THE CANE

Dad was such an independent person.
He never asked for help,
always independent, always in charge.
Now he needs help,
from my sister, from me,
from the assisted living staff.
He can't do it alone anymore,
but he doesn't know how to ask for help.
To him, it's a sign of weakness,
of not fulfilling his promise to Mom,
of not being able to do for her himself.

What a shift for him, for us too.
He was the one we went to when we were in need.
He was the pillar of strength.
Now the pillar of strength is crumbling.
He is getting weaker.
He feels more pain,
both emotionally and physically.
So he is using his cane.
"It helps me to stand up straighter," he tells us.

Will it help him to stand up to what is coming?

BRIDGES

As Mom travels this river of dementia,
she comes to a bridge to her past.
She tries to recall where the bridge goes,
where the bridge came from.
She steps on the bridge,
but cannot remember where it goes.
She steps back into the river of dementia.
After all, it is just water under the bridge.

She cries and doesn't know why.
She can't take the bridge anymore.

Her tears are more water under the bridge.

UNDERCURRENTS

Sometimes there is an undercurrent going on with Mom.
On the surface she tries to hold on to our boat as it moves
with the current.
We look at her and see something else is going on.
Something is flowing beneath the surface, pulling her.
Sometimes the undercurrent is strong
and pulls her away from us.
We cannot swim fast enough to keep her with us.
We see her trying to stay afloat.
We are trying to stay afloat too.

Which one of us will drown first?

OUT OF CONTROL

When she is out of control,
we feel powerless, overwhelmed, helpless.
She explodes, and we implode.

It paralyzes us, to see her out of control.
It's as if the impulse control center of her brain
has opened up,
and she is free of any restraints, any constraints,
no inhibitions, no governing of her behaviors,
her conversations.

Sometimes she opens the door to the unthinkable,
and speaks the unmentionables.
We shut the door to understanding.
We lock ourselves up to feeling.
We exert control over ourselves to counter
her lack of control,
and then we implode.

WAITING FOR THE WELCOMING PARTY

When Mom asked us how we would handle her dying,
I felt her asking me how she would be handling her own death.
I felt some anguish, some worries coming from her.
So I tried to give her comforting words.

I explained about how she would be attending a welcome party,
a party made up of all her family and friends who have gone before her.
I tried to paint a picture of that reunion, that party.
Told her how her parents and brothers
would be at the door,
welcoming her home to her final destination.
I told her God would be waiting to receive her first,
Then the family would be there for her.
I told her I have heard it's very beautiful over there.

"Hey, here comes Mary, hooray, hoorah!" they'd be calling.
They would have open arms and smiles galore,
telling her, "You finally made it home."

I hope that gave her some peace.
I know it gives me peace.

WHO WILL GO FIRST?

Dad has cancer,
Mom has Alzheimer's Disease.
Who will go first?

We have Plan A and Plan B.
If he goes first, we have a plan, Plan A.
She won't be able to fly to NJ and be part of Dad's funeral.
So we have an alternate plan.
Will she know when he goes?
Will she know he's gone?

We'll set up a plan for her to acknowledge his passing,
a service, a ceremony,
a plan to help her understand.
It will all depend on her mental status.
I still feel in some deep level she will understand,
and know that he has gone.
We'll give her the chance to feel, to grieve.
And then we'll move on to our grief.

We can't tell her over and over that Dad has died.
She'll grieve anew each time we tell here.
We'll grieve anew each time we tell her.
But we have to let her grieve,
to feel the pain of his leaving,
to feel the separation, to feel the loss,
to acknowledge the love, the years spent together,

How we tell her will remain a mystery until we do.

PLAN B

Then there is Plan B, if Mom dies first.
Dad will be beside himself with grief.
He will draw strength from us, his children,
his grandchildren,
and whatever family and friends are left.
We will be there to help Dad get through.
We will be there to hold him up, as he holds us up.

We will be there to remember Mom
and all her special gifts.
We will be there to remember their years
of love and devotion,
devotion to each other, to their family and friends,
their faithfulness to each other and faithfulness to God.

Their faith informs them of their future.
They know they will be together again.
We know it too.
That gives us strength to let go
and let God take them home.

It's just that we're not quite ready to let go.

PRACTICING FOR THE FINAL

"What are you going to do when I die?", she asked us.
"How are you girls going to handle things?"
She was concerned about how we would be
after she leaves us.
"Will you be sad and lonely?"
"Will you be lost and hurting?"

Of course we will be all of those things,
lost, hurting, sad, lonely,
missing her for good.

We miss her now,
miss what she used to be,
to us, to Dad.
Can't even imagine what it will feel like when
she is physically gone.
Little by little we lose pieces of her.
Sometimes a light goes on and she returns to us.
But most of the time she is gone,
gone off to some other place, some other time,
traveling on the river of dementia.

Will we be sad and lonely?
Will we be lost and hurting?
You betcha!

We're practicing now.

IS THERE LIFE AFTER CAREGIVING?

I am closing the gap, waiting to retire,
to begin a new part of my life,
explore new directions,
spend time doing what I love.

I've put lots of time in the planning,
the dreaming, the scheming,
mapping out possible routes to take.
I see many roads to take, to travel on.
I look forward to the realization of those dreams.
I have a plan.

What about life after caregiving?
Do we have a plan?
Does Dad, my sister, me?
We've been caregivers so long,
that all the free time,
all the vacation time,
all the 'other' times,
have dealt with caregiving.

We need a plan for after.

HE WENT FIRST

Never expected Dad to go first, not really.
He was always so vigorous in his mind,
even when his body was failing.
He fell, while trying to get to the bathroom.
Hanging on to the bed, the dresser,
he inched his way to the bathroom,
and then his legs gave out and down he went.
He asked Mom to get his cane, but she couldn't help him.
He couldn't even reach the call light.
But he was able to phone my sister and she called for help.
They got him into bed and gave him some pain meds.
Next morning he wasn't able to move and still was in pain.
So he went to the hospital.

It was a long, long wait in the hospital.
My sister sat in the ER for over 10 hours waiting for help.
Our stubborn Father refused pain meds for a long time,
trying to bear the pain, to will it away.
Then the time came when he just couldn't
handle it anymore,
and so he got some relief.
After tests, x-rays and scans they found no breaks.
Checked out if he had Normal Pressure Hydrocephalus.
All the symptoms were there, disorientation,
UTI, gait imbalance.
Oh no, not another parent with mental status changes!
And they wanted us to consider him having
a shunt put in his brain.
Not on a 93 year old man!

We could treat the UTI with antibiotics,
but he would never walk again.
The delirium would probably clear
after the infection cleared.
After talking with his own physician
and checking out the tests,
we discovered it was his spinal stenosis,

a recurrent UTI, and relocation trauma
that was causing the hospitalist to consider
the other diagnosis.

So no brain surgery.
He was up and down during the hospital stay,
sometimes with it, sometimes not.
Whenever I called he was lucid and we chatted.
He was transferred to a Rehab hospital for intensive rehab,
and then he started to go downhill.
I spoke with him Tuesday morning,
asked him if he was coming down with a cold.

He sounded so scratchy voiced and I immediately thought,
pneumonia, he's coming down with pneumonia.
It certainly is possible with someone his age,
lying in bed most of the day.

I told him" Daddy, I love you", he told me he loved me too.
And that was the last time I spoke with him.
That late evening, early morning he went
into respiratory distress.
My sister got the call from the hospital that
he needed help to breathe.
So we put him on a Bi-Pap machine
to see if it would help him breathe long enough,
hoping the antibiotics would kick in.
My sister and I were in constant phone conversation,
back and forth with the hospital, with Dad's physician,
with each other.
We decided to put him on a ventilator for 2-3 days,
again hoping the antibiotics would kick in.
Then we would decide the next step.

Christmas came and went.
We all tried to make some special times with our families.
We were with our children and grandchildren almost
3,000 miles away.
We could not fly to South Carolina,
as the country was hit with major blizzards
in the mid-west.
We found we couldn't get to Charleston.

Couldn't even get home to Wyoming
due to the blizzard there.
So we waited it out, surrounded
by our children and grandchildren.
Every time the phone rang there were
major crises to discuss.

My sister handled everything.
Her husband and her daughter were there with her,
and then her son flew in from Boston
to say goodbye to Grandpa.
My children and I said goodbye by telephone.
But I really said good bye at my last visit to Mom and Dad.
I remember Dad holding on to me very tightly,
as I hugged him good bye.
I told him I would see him soon,
and he said, "I don't' think so."
I felt at that time it was the last good bye.
So I was ready to let Dad go.

But we still needed some time to give the drugs
a chance to work,

And for us to talk about the possibility of his dying,
and what to do next.
We waited until the day after Christmas
to take him off the vent.
My sister, her husband and children
were at the hospital by his side.
I was on the phone connected to them and ready.
He did not die immediately.
That strong hearted and stubborn Hungarian man
fought to stay.
He held on for 12 more hours
and then went in the middle of the night.
My sister had gone home to sleep
when she got the call to come back.
He died before she got there at 3:12 am on December 27.

On the phone we all listened to my husband,
a retired minister, pray.
His prayer was for Dad and us, reminding us of Dad's faith,

of his completing his journey,
and a prayer for all of us coping with Dad's passing,
coping with our loss.
But mostly it was about celebration,
celebrating Dad's arrival at his new home,
and celebrating our faith and hope.

My sister signed the papers, called the funeral home,
made the plans we decided on for Dad
Then she went home for sleep.
And so did we all sleep.

My sister then went to Mom's place to tell her
Dad was gone.
Mom didn't get it.
My sister kept Mom informed that Dad was very sick
and might die.
Mom didn't get it then.
My sister told her Dad had died and gone to heaven.
Mom didn't get it now.
But she did ask my sister
when Dad was coming home from work.
After several more times my sister
finally got through to Mom.
Mom said she was sad about losing Dad
and cried a little bit too.
But then moved on to other tidbits of conversation.

So now we know she can't process the information.
When she asks about Dad we'll tell her
he's waiting for her at his new place,
that he's getting it ready for her when she comes,
and that it won't be long.
Good grief, I hope it's not long.
I hope they will be reunited soon,
and both will be at their journey's end,
the end of traveling on the river of dementia.

We are making plans to fly to South Carolina
after we fly home to Wyoming.
Have to renew prescriptions, pay bills, book a flight,
do laundry, get someone to watch the horses and house,

and drive 3 hours to Denver, New Year's Eve
to get an early flight.
I need to see my sister, grieve with her together.
I need to see where my Father's ashes are held.

And I need to help my sister empty my father's apartment.
On Monday a new resident moves in.
So we have our work cut out for us.
Cleaning out the old place, sorting through his stuff,
meeting with the lawyer, the banker trust officer,
the funeral director,
planning Dad's memorial service together,
sorting through photos for a photo essay of his life,
meeting with Mom to help her understand,
to help her know that Dad is planning a reunion soon,
and they will be together forever.

He's completed his journey, his walk.
We are the ones, my sister and me,
the ones left to accompany Mom on her travels,
along the river of dementia.

We won't let you down, Dad.

FINAL JOURNEY

Dad was always on the move,
planes, trains, automobiles, walking.
How he loved to travel, to see new things,
to explore and enjoy,
whether it was trips to Hawaii, to Europe, to the
Caribbean,
all over the USA,
or trips to visit the kids and grandkids.
How he loved to travel,
especially the open road.
Oh the stories we can tell about our road trips!

Now he has embarked on his final journey.
He's going home.
(He'll still be checking out the places for Mom
to come and see when it's her turn.)

As he got closer to his final destination,
he slowed down a bit,
knowing it was coming soon.
He had a shuffle in his walk,
taking his time,
taking it all in,
savoring the last walks,
taking time to stop, take a breath and take it all in,
and say goodbye.

His whole life he had been wrapped in God's arms.
a man of faith, a man of love,
a man of honor, a man of integrity.
His prayer was "Whenever you call, Lord, I am ready."
He was ready.

So we let him go.
We gave him the gift to go.
We were just prolonging his journey, for our sakes.
So we let him go.

He is at home in his eternal home.

Now we receive the gifts from God.
The gifts of faith that assures us we'll be together again.
The gifts of love in knowing how much we were
loved and cherished,
and will continue to be loved.
The gift of joy in knowing he is at peace with God
and that God will give us God's peace.
The gift of release knowing his pain is over
and his final destination has arrived.

Goodbye Dad.
Goodbye Grandpa,
Goodbye Great-Grandpa
Goodbye from your beloved wife, Mary.

We loved you so much.
We're sending you home
Your journey is over.

Amen and Amen.

FINAL GOODBYE

I said goodbye on Tuesday morning,
told him I loved him and he told me he loved me too.
He was in the hospital for a while after his fall,
in lots of pain.
He couldn't walk.
The therapists tried and it was not going to happen.
I think when he knew he couldn't walk,
his walk was over.
The time that he could take charge of his life,
determine how to go about things,
was over.
His walk was truly over.

So he lay down in bed and gave his body over.
With being bedridden the pneumonia took charge.
He was too weak to breathe on his own
and to allow the antibiotics to work.
We decided to give his body a break
and let the ventilator help him breathe.

My sister told him to relax,
and said "I'm going to take care of you, Daddy,
I'm going to take care of Mommy, too."
His breathing that was previously labored and heavy,
became relaxed.
He heard.

After a few days we knew he was going home.
We were just prolonging his journey, for our sakes.
So we let him go.
Onward, upward, now walking,
now running to his final home.

Good bye Dad.
We loved you so much.
We're sending you home.

SIX YEARS LATER

Six years after our Dad died, Mom joined him.
Those six years we watched her plateau
and then slowly fade away.
She had mostly disappeared into dementia.
We continued to visit the shell of her former self.
Yes, she was still our Mother and we were her daughters.
And we visited.

The disease that ate away at her personality,
her uniqueness,
began to erode her frail body.
It was painful to see her body's outer shell.
She was now 98 years, 6 months old.
My sister has moved to Florida for her retirement,
and to be near her daughter and family.
My husband had died from cancer a year
after my Dad passed.
Our lives had changed.

But Mom continued to hold on to life.
We learned patience during those six years,
and we tried to model for our children
how to provide care for elderly parents,
how to love and remember the joys of a life well lived.

What a gift we had in having Mom for almost 99 years,
and Dad for 93 years.

Our journey on the River of Dementia was finally over.

IT'S OVER

It's over. The long good bye has finally come to an end. She has truly left us. At 4:39 on November 11 she danced off to heaven. Sunday we got a call from her nursing home that she was failing. So we alerted our families that Grandmom was getting ready to go. We expected her to die that night but she plateaued and hung on to life for a few more days, giving us a chance to accept her passing.

My nephew was able to be with her for a bit the night before she died. She took some nourishment for the body, a bit of baby food to eat. And a bit of nourishment for the soul. When my nephew squeezed her hand, she squeezed back, acknowledging his presence. How we wanted her to acknowledge our presence whenever we visited her this last year. She mentally left us a long time ago. Yet during my last visit she beamed at me in recognition and then cried when I left, acknowledging she knew who I was.

Now I smile, beam and cry at her joining with Dad, her departed family as she makes the final journey to her eternal home. She is at peace and may we be at peace, envisioning her waltzing into Dad's arms.

I have just returned from a trip to the Danube, traveling to some of the same places she and Dad had visited - Vienna and Budapest. I took loads of pictures hoping that when I visited her at Thanksgiving, they would trigger a memory for her. How calmly and peacefully the Danube river flowed. No turbulence, nor rocks to steer around, no rapids to avoid. For that has been the story of Mom's journey on the river of dementia, filled with turbulence, rocks to steer around and rapids to avoid. The Danube has locks along its river course to avoid all those dangers, the rapids, the turbulence, to ease the passing over the rugged waterways.

Eventually the turbulence in my Mother's mind was locked out and she was able to sail smoothly at last over the river of dementia and into the next step in the river of time. Her journey on the river of dementia is over. May she be at peace. May we be at peace. Amen and Amen.

WHEN IT'S OVER

The river of dementia flows into the sea,
joins with all the other rivers.
The great river becomes the womb of a new life,
a baptism into life after this life.
We hope we will all be united in that baptism into new life.

I plan to have my ashes strewn over the ocean,
reuniting with the waters of life,
waters of my Mother's womb,
waters of my own baptism,
waters of my own being,
reuniting me with all who have traveled the river of life,
reuniting with those special ones,
who have traveled on the river of dementia.

May we all be free and pure,
and be joyful in the calm after the final surge.
May our journey on the river of dementia be complete.

THE RIVER OF TIME

Rivers bisect the landscape,
joining with the ribbon,
adding to the flow,
like families
flowing on a course through the landscape of life,
welcoming new members into the flow.

Never a straight path,
but one that meanders, mossies, rushes,
twists, turns.
How unique to see it from the air,
like a map.
Can't see the beginning or the end.
Like families,
it continues to flow,
going where it will.

We enter the river of life,
embraced by family,
who guide us, guard us, love us,
swimming with us on the river.
Sometimes we stop on the way,
sometimes we wade in,
sometimes we plunge in,
not knowing where the river will take us.
We say goodbye to some,
hello to others.

The river goes on.
It keeps on,
and we keep on,
empowered by those who bore us on the river,
who leave us on the river,
and say, - "Go" –
keep on for us.

We live in you,
We flow in you.
flowing with you.

www.ingramcontent.com/pod-product-compliance
Lightning Source LLC
Chambersburg PA
CBHW020540030426
42337CB00013B/916